## Disclaimer

This book is intended for informational purposes only and is not a substitute for professional medical advice, diagnosis, or treatment. The content provided herein is based on research, personal experiences, and anecdotal evidence related to pH balance and nutrition. The information in this book is not medical advice in any way. Contact your medical or health care provide for any health related questions, issue.

While every effort has been made to ensure the accuracy and completeness of the information, the field of nutrition and health is continuously evolving, and new findings may alter some of the concepts and recommendations presented. The publisher or author is not responsible for any errors or omissions.

Readers are advised to consult with a qualified healthcare professional before making any significant changes to their diet or lifestyle, especially if they have pre-existing health conditions, are pregnant, nursing, or taking medication. The author and publisher are not responsible for any adverse effects or consequences resulting from the use of any of the suggestions, preparations, or procedures discussed in this book.

The dietary and lifestyle choices described in this book are not intended as a one-size-fits-all approach. Individual nutritional needs and health concerns vary, and what may be beneficial for one person may not be suitable for another. Therefore, readers should tailor the information to their unique circumstances and health objectives.

By using the information in this book, the reader agrees to assume full responsibility for any risks or adverse effects that may arise. The author and publisher disclaim any liability, loss, or risk, personal or otherwise, which is incurred as a direct or indirect consequence of the use or application of any of the contents of this book. This information or statements in this educational book have not been evaluated by the Food and Drug Administration. This information is not intended to diagnose, treat, cure, or prevent any disease

**About Traverse Bay Farms:**

Since 2009, Traverse Bay Farms has won 38+ national food awards at America's largest and most competitive food competitions. In addition to offering a nationally award-winning cherry-based products, here is a brief overview of their additional award-winning products and all-natural products:

Cherry Juice Concentrate – 100% Pure Montmorency Cherry Juice Concentrate

Salsas:

- Cherry
- Black Bean
- Corn
- Red Raspberry
- Mango
- Pineapple
- Garlic
- Bacon

Jams and Butters:

- Bacon Jam
- Blueberry Jam
- Monkey Butter
- Apple Butter
- Pumpkin Butter

Dried Fruit:

- Cherries (Organic)
- Blueberries (Organic)
- Apples
- Strawberries

Fruit Powders:

- Cherry (Organic)
- Blueberry (Organic)

## Fruit Supplements:

- Tart Cherry Joint Formula
- Wild Blueberry Brain Support
- Pomegranate Heart Health
- Raspberry Ketone Weight Management
- Cherry Prime – Patented Formula

## Salad Dressings, Beets and Maple Syrup:

- Cherry Poppyseed
- Strawberry Poppyseed
- Maple Vinaigrette
- Blueberry Balsamic Vinaigrette
- Michigan Maple Syrup
- Cinnamon Pickled Baby Beets

## Barbecue Sauces

- Cherry
- Red Raspberry
- Apple

## Contents

## Introduction

This book embarks on an enlightening journey into the fascinating world of dietary pH and its profound impact on our health and well-being. The concept of acidity and alkalinity in the human body is more than just a fleeting health trend; it's a pivotal aspect of understanding how our dietary choices influence our physical state.

The human body operates optimally within a delicate balance of acidity and alkalinity. This balance, known as the pH level, is a critical factor that affects various physiological processes. The foods we eat play a significant role in maintaining this balance, affecting our health in ways we often overlook. In this guide, we delve into the science of pH, unraveling how it works in our bodies and the effects of different foods on our overall pH balance.

Our exploration begins with a clear, concise explanation of what constitutes acidic and alkaline foods. We'll debunk common myths and shine a light on the factual science behind the body's pH regulation. Understanding the intricate relationship between diet and body pH is crucial, as it lays the foundation for making informed dietary choices.

Throughout this book, we present a balanced view, acknowledging that while extreme diets are not the answer, thoughtful consideration of the acidity or alkalinity of foods can contribute significantly to our health. Whether you're looking to make minor adjustments to your diet or seeking a comprehensive understanding of pH balance in nutrition, this guide offers valuable insights, practical advice, and evidence-based information to help you on your journey to optimal health.

Join us as we navigate the complexities of acidity and alkaline foods, and learn how to harmonize your diet with your body's natural needs, paving the way for a healthier, more vibrant life.

## The Science of pH in the Human Body

### Understanding pH balance

The concept of pH balance is fundamental to both chemistry and biology, playing a crucial role in various aspects of human health. In simple terms, pH (potential of hydrogen) measures the acidity or alkalinity of a substance on a scale ranging from 0 to 14. A pH of 7 is considered neutral, as in pure water. Values below 7 indicate acidity, while values above 7 indicate alkalinity.

### The Significance of pH in the Human Body

The human body is a complex system, requiring a specific and delicate pH balance to function optimally. Different parts of the body have different pH levels; for example, stomach acid is highly acidic with a pH around 2, essential for food digestion, whereas blood is slightly alkaline, with a normal pH range of 7.35 to 7.45.

Maintaining the pH balance in the blood is vital. Even minor deviations can disrupt cellular functions and metabolic processes, leading to health complications. The body employs various mechanisms to regulate its pH, including the respiratory system, the kidneys, and buffer systems in the blood.

### Respiratory Regulation of pH

The respiratory system helps maintain pH balance by controlling the levels of carbon dioxide ($CO_2$) in the blood. $CO_2$ is slightly acidic, and its concentration is directly linked to the pH of the blood. When $CO_2$ levels rise, the blood becomes more acidic, and the respiratory system responds by increasing breathing rate to expel more $CO_2$. Conversely, if $CO_2$ levels drop, the breathing rate slows down, increasing the blood's acidity.

### Renal Regulation of pH

The kidneys also play a vital role in regulating body pH. They do this by excreting or retaining hydrogen ions ($H^+$) and bicarbonate ions ($HCO_3^-$) in the urine. When the blood is too acidic, the kidneys excrete more $H^+$ and retain $HCO_3^-$, helping to raise the pH back to normal. In the case of alkaline blood, the process reverses.

## Buffer Systems

Buffer systems in the blood are another line of defense against pH imbalance. These systems consist of weak acids and their corresponding bases, which work together to minimize pH changes. The most significant buffer system in human blood involves carbonic acid ($H_2CO_3$) and bicarbonate ($HCO_3^-$). This system can neutralize excess acids or bases, keeping the blood pH within its narrow range.

## Diet and Body pH

The role of diet in influencing body pH has been a topic of much discussion and research. While it's a common belief that consuming certain foods can significantly alter the body's overall pH, the truth is more nuanced. The body's buffering systems efficiently maintain pH balance regardless of dietary intake. However, long-term consumption of highly acidic or alkaline foods can strain these regulatory systems, potentially leading to health issues over time.

Acidic foods, such as meat, dairy, and processed foods, can increase the body's acid load, whereas alkaline foods like fruits and vegetables help balance this effect. It's essential to note that the acidity or alkalinity of foods refers to their ash residue after digestion, not their actual pH.

## Conclusion

Understanding pH balance is key to appreciating how our bodies function and the impact of our diet on overall health. While the body is remarkably adept at maintaining pH balance, our dietary choices can influence its efficiency. A balanced diet, rich in a variety of nutrients, helps support the body's natural regulatory mechanisms, promoting health and preventing imbalances that could lead to disease. This chapter sets the stage for a deeper exploration of acidic and alkaline foods and their effects on the body, which we will delve into in the following chapters.

## Importance of pH in health and disease

The pH level of our body plays a critical role in maintaining health and preventing disease. This delicate balance, often taken for granted, is a cornerstone of our physiological well-being. In this chapter, we explore the profound impact of pH on various aspects of health and how imbalances can lead to disease.

### pH and Disease Prevention

A balanced pH level is essential for the normal functioning of cells and organs. The body's natural pH balance helps in the efficient transport of nutrients and removal of waste, optimal enzyme function, and proper immune response. When this balance is disrupted, it can lead to a range of health issues.

### Chronic Acidosis and Health Risks

Chronic acidosis, a condition where the body's pH tilts towards acidity over an extended period, has been linked to several health problems. This condition can be caused by poor diet, certain medications, chronic respiratory issues, or kidney problems. Studies have shown that chronic acidosis may contribute to:

1. **Osteoporosis**: The body may leach calcium from bones to neutralize excess acid, potentially weakening bones over time.
2. **Muscle Degradation**: Acidic environments can lead to muscle wasting, as the body may break down muscle tissue to free up amino acids for use in pH regulation.
3. **Kidney Stones**: An acidic environment in the kidneys can lead to the formation of certain types of kidney stones.
4. **Increased Cardiovascular Risk**: Some research suggests that acidosis can increase inflammation and stress on the cardiovascular system.

### Alkalosis and its Effects

Alkalosis, the opposite condition where the body is too alkaline, is less common but can be equally harmful. It often results from excessive vomiting, diuretic use, or hormonal imbalances. Alkalosis can lead to:

1. **Electrolyte Imbalance**: Disruption in electrolyte levels can affect muscle and nerve function.
2. **Decreased Calcium**: High pH can bind calcium, making it less available for bodily functions, potentially leading to muscle spasms and tetany.

## Dietary Influence on pH and Health

While the body tightly regulates its pH, diet can still play a role, particularly in the context of chronic dietary habits. A diet high in acidic foods (like meat, dairy, and processed foods) can increase the body's acid load. Conversely, alkaline diets, rich in fruits and vegetables, can help balance this effect.

## pH in Digestive Health

The pH levels in the digestive system are particularly important. For example, the stomach requires a highly acidic environment to break down food effectively. Conversely, the intestines need a more neutral environment. Disruptions in these pH levels can lead to digestive issues like acid reflux, ulcers, or poor nutrient absorption.

## The Role of pH in Cancer

Research into the relationship between pH and cancer is ongoing. Some studies suggest that cancer cells thrive in acidic environments and that an alkaline diet might slow cancer growth. However, these claims require more scientific validation, as the body's buffering systems generally maintain a stable pH, regardless of dietary intake.

## Conclusion

Understanding the role of pH in health and disease is vital for maintaining overall well-being. While the body has robust mechanisms to regulate its pH, chronic imbalances, often influenced by diet and lifestyle, can have significant health implications. By acknowledging the importance of pH balance, individuals can make informed choices about their diet and lifestyle, potentially reducing the risk of pH-related health issues. The next chapters will further explore how specific dietary choices can impact the body's pH and overall health.

## Overview of Acidity and Alkalinity in Foods

### How foods influence body's pH

Understanding the influence of diet on the body's pH is crucial for maintaining optimal health. While the human body has a remarkable capacity to regulate its internal pH, the foods we consume can significantly affect this balance. In this chapter, we'll explore how different foods impact the body's pH and specifically examine the benefits of cherry-based foods like cherry juice and dried cherries.

### Acidic and Alkaline Foods

Foods are categorized as acidic or alkaline based on their potential renal acid load (PRAL) and their effect on the body's pH after metabolism, not necessarily their inherent pH. When metabolized, acidic foods can increase the body's acid load, potentially straining the body's buffering systems. Common acidic foods include meat, dairy products, eggs, and processed grains. On the other hand, alkaline foods, predominantly fruits and vegetables, can help neutralize this acidity.

### Role of Cherries in pH Balance

Cherries, particularly in the form of cherry juice and dried cherries, are an excellent example of how certain foods can benefit the body's pH balance. Cherries are rich in antioxidants, vitamins, and minerals and have an alkalizing effect on the body. This effect makes them particularly beneficial for counteracting the acidity from a diet high in animal proteins and processed foods.

**Health Benefits of Cherry Juice and Dried Cherries**

1. **Anti-Inflammatory Properties**: Cherries are renowned for their anti-inflammatory effects, attributed to their high antioxidant content, including anthocyanins and flavonoids. These compounds help reduce inflammation and can alleviate conditions like arthritis and gout.
2. **Muscle Recovery and Pain Relief**: Studies have shown that cherry juice can aid in muscle recovery post-exercise. The antioxidants in cherries help reduce muscle damage and pain, making cherry juice a popular choice among athletes.
3. **Improved Sleep Quality**: Cherries, particularly tart cherries, contain natural melatonin, a hormone that regulates the sleep-wake cycle. Consuming cherry juice or dried cherries can help improve sleep quality and duration.
4. **Cardiovascular Health**: The potassium and polyphenol content in cherries can help lower blood pressure and reduce the risk of cardiovascular diseases. They aid in maintaining a healthy balance of electrolytes, crucial for heart function.
5. **Digestive Health**: Cherries have a moderate fiber content, especially in their dried form, which aids in digestion and promotes a healthy gut. This fiber also assists in maintaining a stable blood sugar level.
6. **Alkalizing Effect**: By contributing to a more alkaline environment in the body, cherries can help neutralize the acidic effects of other foods, promoting overall pH balance and reducing the risk of acid-related health issues.

**Incorporating Cherries into the Diet**

Incorporating cherries into the diet is simple and beneficial. Cherry juice can be consumed as a refreshing drink, preferably without added sugars to maintain its health properties. Dried cherries can be added to oatmeal, yogurt, or salads, or enjoyed as a healthy snack. It's important to note that while cherries are beneficial, they should be part of a balanced diet that includes a variety of fruits and vegetables.

**Conclusion**

The impact of diet on the body's pH is a nuanced but important aspect of nutrition. While the body efficiently regulates its pH, the foods we consume can influence this balance.

Cherry-based foods, like cherry juice and dried cherries, offer a plethora of health benefits, from reducing inflammation and aiding in muscle recovery to improving sleep and promoting cardiovascular health. By understanding how different foods affect the body's pH, individuals can make informed dietary choices that support overall health and well-being. The next chapter will delve deeper into the ways to measure and balance dietary pH for optimal health.

## Myths and facts

The world of nutrition is often clouded by myths, especially regarding the effects of diet on the body's pH balance. In this chapter, we aim to clarify these misconceptions by separating myths from facts, providing a clearer understanding of how acidity and alkalinity truly impact our health.

### Myth 1: The Body's pH Can Be Significantly Altered by Diet

*Fact*: While diet can influence the pH of urine, it has little effect on blood pH, which is tightly regulated by the body. The human body has evolved robust mechanisms, including the respiratory and renal systems, to maintain the blood's pH within a very narrow range. Extreme dietary changes are unlikely to have a significant impact on this tightly regulated system.

### Myth 2: Acidic Foods Are Harmful and Should Be Avoided

*Fact*: Acidic foods, such as citrus fruits, are not harmful to health; in fact, they are rich in essential nutrients and antioxidants. The idea that these foods acidify the body is a misunderstanding. For instance, lemon and lime, although acidic in nature, have an alkalizing effect after digestion. The key is balance and moderation in the diet.

### Myth 3: Alkaline Diets Can Cure Cancer

*Fact*: There is no scientific evidence to support the claim that alkaline diets can cure cancer. Cancer cells can grow in both acidic and alkaline environments. While a balanced diet rich in fruits and vegetables can support overall health and may reduce the risk of many types of cancer, it is not a standalone cure.

### Myth 4: High-Protein Diets Cause Acidosis and Bone Loss

*Fact*: High-protein diets, especially those rich in animal proteins, can increase the acid load in the body. However, in healthy individuals, the kidneys efficiently excrete this excess acid. While there were concerns about bone loss due to calcium leaching to neutralize the acid, recent studies indicate that protein intake is also associated with better bone health, likely due to its role in bone formation and maintenance.

### Myth 5: Drinking Alkaline Water Leads to Better Health

*Fact*: Alkaline water has a higher pH level than regular drinking water. While some proponents claim health benefits like anti-aging properties, improved metabolism, and cancer resistance, these claims lack substantial scientific backing. For most people, drinking regular water is sufficient to maintain hydration and health.

## Myth 6: Acid Reflux is Caused Solely by Acidic Foods

*Fact*: Acid reflux is a complex condition that can be triggered by various factors, including overeating, obesity, certain medications, and a weakened lower esophageal sphincter. While acidic foods can exacerbate symptoms in some individuals, they are not the sole cause of acid reflux.

## Myth 7: Urine pH is a Reliable Indicator of Overall Health

*Fact*: While urine pH can reflect recent dietary intake, it is not a reliable indicator of overall health or the body's internal pH balance. Urine pH can vary significantly throughout the day based on numerous factors, including food and fluid intake.

## Conclusion

Understanding the myths and facts about diet, acidity, and alkalinity is crucial for making informed nutritional choices. While the principles of acidic and alkaline foods can guide healthier eating habits, it's essential to approach this topic with a balanced perspective. A varied diet rich in fruits, vegetables, whole grains, and lean proteins, coupled with regular physical activity, remains the cornerstone of good health. The next chapter will focus on evaluating and balancing your diet for optimal pH and overall health.

## Chapter 1: The Basics of Acidic and Alkaline Foods

### Defining Acidic and Alkaline Foods

In the quest to understand the impact of diet on health, the concepts of acidic and alkaline foods have garnered significant attention. This chapter aims to provide a scientific explanation of what constitutes acidic and alkaline foods, and how they are defined in the context of human nutrition.

### The Concept of pH in Foods

At its core, the classification of foods into acidic or alkaline categories is based on the concept of pH. pH is a scale that measures the acidity or alkalinity of a substance, ranging from 0 (highly acidic) to 14 (highly alkaline), with 7 being neutral. However, when it comes to foods, the determination of acidity or alkalinity is not as straightforward as measuring their pH levels.

### Potential Renal Acid Load (PRAL)

The classification of foods as acidic or alkaline in nutrition is primarily based on their Potential Renal Acid Load (PRAL). PRAL is a measure of the production of acid or alkali in the kidneys after the body metabolizes the food. This concept is crucial because it reflects the effect of food on the body's internal environment, rather than its inherent pH level.

### Acidic Foods

Acidic foods are those that contribute to an increase in the body's acid load. This doesn't necessarily mean these foods are acidic in nature; rather, they produce acid upon digestion and metabolism. These foods typically include:

1. **Animal Proteins**: Meat, poultry, fish, and eggs tend to have high PRAL values, meaning they increase acid production.
2. **Grains and Processed Foods**: Most grains, like wheat and rice, and processed foods are acid-forming due to their protein and phosphorus content.
3. **Dairy Products**: Cheese, milk, and other dairy products also contribute to an acidic environment in the body.

## Alkaline Foods

Alkaline foods, on the other hand, are those that reduce the acid load in the body. They are typically rich in potassium and magnesium, which are alkaline minerals. Alkaline foods generally include:

1. **Fruits and Vegetables**: Most fruits and vegetables are alkaline-forming. They are high in minerals that neutralize acids.
2. **Nuts and Seeds**: Many nuts and seeds also have alkaline-forming properties.
3. **Legumes**: Beans, lentils, and other legumes can contribute to an alkaline environment in the body.

## The Role of Minerals in Determining Food Acidity

The acid or alkaline-forming nature of foods is largely influenced by their mineral content. Foods rich in calcium, magnesium, and potassium tend to be alkaline-forming, while those high in phosphorus, sulfur, and chloride are generally acid-forming.

## The Ash Residue Concept

The classification into acidic or alkaline also derives from the concept of 'ash residue.' This refers to the residue left after a food is completely burned, which indicates the type of minerals predominant in the food. If the ash is high in alkaline minerals, the food is considered alkaline, and vice versa.

## Conclusion

Understanding the scientific basis of acidic and alkaline foods requires a shift from traditional pH measurement to a focus on the metabolic end products of these foods in the body. The balance between acidic and alkaline foods in the diet is key to maintaining good health. This understanding paves the way for subsequent chapters that delve into the impacts of diet on body pH, and how to create a balanced and nutritious dietary plan.

## Common acidic and alkaline foods

A balanced diet requires an understanding of the foods that contribute to the body's acid and alkaline load. This chapter provides an extensive list of common acidic and alkaline foods, including the roles of dried cherries, cherry juice, blueberries, and dried blueberries.

## Acidic Foods

Acidic foods, when metabolized, contribute to an increase in the body's acid load. It's important to note that the acidity of a food item isn't determined by its initial pH but by the type of residue it leaves in the body after digestion.

- **Animal Proteins**:
  - Red meat, poultry, fish
  - Processed meats like sausages and deli meats
- **Dairy Products**:
  - Milk, cheese, yogurt, and butter
- **Grains and Cereals**:
  - Wheat, oats, rice, and rye
  - Bread, pasta, and breakfast cereals
- **Processed and Sugary Foods**:
  - Candies, cookies, cakes, and other sweet treats
  - Soft drinks and sweetened beverages
- **Caffeinated Beverages and Alcohol**:
  - Coffee, tea (especially black tea)
  - Alcoholic drinks like beer, wine, and spirits

## Alkaline Foods

Alkaline foods help to neutralize the body's acid load. These are predominantly fruits, vegetables, nuts, and seeds, rich in alkaline minerals like potassium, calcium, and magnesium.

- **Fruits**:
  - Citrus fruits like lemons and oranges (despite their acidic nature)
  - Melons such as watermelon and cantaloupe
  - Tropical fruits like mangoes, papayas, and pineapples
  - **Cherries and Blueberries**:
    - **Dried Cherries**: Packed with antioxidants, dried cherries have an alkalizing effect on the body. They are also rich in vitamins and fiber.
    - **Cherry Juice**: Fresh cherry juice is another alkaline option. It retains most of the nutrients and antioxidants of fresh cherries and contributes to reducing the body's acid load.
    - **Blueberries**: Fresh or frozen, they are an alkaline-forming fruit. Blueberries are high in antioxidants and vitamins.
    - **Dried Blueberries**: Similar to dried cherries, dried blueberries are an alkaline food choice, offering a convenient and nutrient-dense snack.
- **Vegetables**:
  - Leafy greens like spinach, kale, and Swiss chard
  - Cruciferous vegetables such as broccoli, cauliflower, and Brussels sprouts
  - Root vegetables like sweet potatoes and carrots
- **Nuts and Seeds**:
  - Almonds, chia seeds, flaxseeds
  - Pumpkin seeds and sunflower seeds
- **Legumes**:
  - Beans (black beans, kidney beans, etc.)
  - Lentils and chickpeas
- **Others**:
  - Tofu and other soy products
  - Herbal teas

## The Role of Acidic and Alkaline Foods in the Diet

Incorporating a balance of acidic and alkaline foods is crucial for maintaining good health. While it's not necessary to completely avoid acidic foods, being mindful of their consumption and balancing them with alkaline foods is beneficial.

- **Moderation with Acidic Foods**:
  - Consume animal proteins and dairy in moderation.
  - Opt for whole grains over processed cereals and bread.
  - Limit intake of sugary and processed foods, as well as caffeine and alcohol.
- **Emphasizing Alkaline Foods**:
  - Increase the intake of fruits and vegetables.
  - Include nuts and seeds as part of a balanced diet.
  - Choose legumes as a plant-based protein source.
  - Hydrate with water and herbal teas instead of sugary drinks.

## Health Benefits of a Balanced pH Diet

Consuming a diet that balances acidic and alkaline foods has several health benefits:

- **Bone Health**: A diet rich in alkaline fruits and vegetables can help in maintaining strong bones.
- **Muscle Mass**: Alkaline diets may help in preserving muscle mass as we age.
- **Cardiovascular Health**: Foods like blueberries and cherries have been linked to improved heart health due to their antioxidant properties.
- **Digestive Wellness**: Alkaline foods, particularly high-fiber fruits and vegetables, promote healthy digestion.
- **Overall Well-being**: A balanced pH diet supports overall health and can help in preventing chronic diseases.

## Conclusion

Understanding and incorporating a mix of acidic and alkaline foods, including nutrient-rich options like dried cherries, cherry juice, blueberries, and dried blueberries, can significantly contribute to a well-rounded, healthful diet. This balance is not about completely eliminating certain food groups but about creating a dietary harmony that supports the body's

**How the Body Regulates pH**

**The Role of Kidneys, Lungs, and Other Organs in pH Balance**

The human body is a remarkable system that maintains a stable internal environment, including the pH level, through the coordinated work of various organs. The kidneys and lungs play a primary role in this regulation, but the liver, intestines, and lymphatic system also contribute significantly. This chapter explores the functions of these organs in maintaining the body's pH balance.

**Kidneys: Masters of Chemical Balance**

The kidneys are crucial in regulating the body's pH by controlling the balance of acids and bases. They perform this task through several mechanisms:

1. **Excretion of Hydrogen Ions**: The kidneys remove excess hydrogen ions (H+) from the body through urine. This process is essential for neutralizing acidity.
2. **Reabsorption and Production of Bicarbonate**: Bicarbonate (HCO3-) is a base that neutralizes acids. The kidneys not only reabsorb bicarbonate from the urine but also produce new bicarbonate to replace what is used to neutralize acids in the body.
3. **Excretion of Acidic and Alkaline Salts**: The kidneys regulate the excretion of acidic and alkaline compounds. This fine-tuning helps maintain the delicate balance of the body's pH.

**Lungs: Regulating Acid-Base Balance Through Respiration**

The lungs contribute to pH balance by regulating carbon dioxide (CO2) levels in the blood, which is intrinsically linked to pH. The process includes:

1. **Removal of Carbon Dioxide**: CO2 is a byproduct of cellular metabolism and is carried in the blood to the lungs. When CO2 levels are high, it increases the acidity of the blood. The lungs help by exhaling CO2, thus reducing acidity.
2. **Respiratory Rate Adjustment**: The body can adjust the respiratory rate to maintain pH balance. If blood becomes too acidic, breathing becomes faster and deeper to expel more CO2. Conversely, if the blood is too alkaline, breathing slows to retain CO2.

## Liver: Metabolic Regulation and Detoxification

The liver, while not directly involved in pH regulation, plays a supportive role:

1. **Metabolism of Amino Acids**: The liver metabolizes amino acids, which can produce acids or bases. The liver's efficient processing of these compounds helps in maintaining overall metabolic balance.
2. **Detoxification**: The liver neutralizes toxins, which could otherwise alter the body's pH if they accumulated.

## Intestines: Acid-Base Balance Through Bicarbonate Secretion

The role of the intestines in pH balance is often overlooked:

1. **Secretion of Bicarbonate**: The pancreas (a part of the digestive system) secretes bicarbonate into the small intestine, which neutralizes stomach acid and creates an optimal pH for digestive enzymes.

## Lymphatic System: Maintaining Tissue pH

The lymphatic system helps maintain tissue fluid pH by draining excess fluids and proteins from tissues and returning them to the bloodstream. This process includes:

1. **Fluid Balance**: By regulating the fluid balance in tissues, the lymphatic system helps prevent the local environment from becoming too acidic or too alkaline.
2. **Immune Function**: The lymphatic system is also crucial for immune function, which can be affected by pH changes.

## Conclusion

The body's ability to maintain pH balance is a testament to the intricate interplay of various organ systems. The kidneys and lungs are at the forefront of this regulation, but the liver, intestines, and lymphatic system also play vital roles. Understanding these mechanisms highlights the importance of maintaining the health of these organs for optimal pH balance and overall well-being. The next chapter will explore the long-term effects of an acidic diet on the body and its systems.

## Buffer systems in the body

The human body operates in a delicate balance, constantly adjusting to maintain a stable internal environment, or homeostasis. One of the critical aspects of this balance is pH regulation. The body's buffer systems play a crucial role in maintaining the pH within a narrow range, essential for various physiological processes. This chapter delves into the intricacies of these buffer systems, their components, and their functions.

## Understanding Buffer Systems

A buffer system is a mixture of a weak acid and its conjugate base (or a weak base and its conjugate acid) that can resist changes in pH. When an acid (donates hydrogen ions, H+) or a base (accepts hydrogen ions) is added to the system, the buffer solution can absorb these excess ions, maintaining a relatively stable pH.

## Key Buffer Systems in the Body

1. **Bicarbonate Buffer System**:
   - The primary buffer system in the blood.
   - Composed of bicarbonate ion ($HCO_3-$) as the base and carbonic acid ($H_2CO_3$) as the acid.
   - When pH rises, carbonic acid dissociates to release hydrogen ions (H+), lowering the pH.
   - Conversely, when pH falls, bicarbonate ions trap excess hydrogen ions, increasing the pH.
   - This buffer system works in tandem with the lungs and kidneys. The lungs regulate the concentration of carbon dioxide ($CO_2$), and the kidneys regulate bicarbonate concentration.
2. **Phosphate Buffer System**:
   - Predominantly functions in the kidneys and intracellular fluids.
   - Comprises dihydrogen phosphate ($H_2PO_4-$) as the acid and hydrogen phosphate ($HPO_4^{2-}$) as the base.
   - Plays a vital role in the renal handling of hydrogen ions.
3. **Protein Buffer Systems**:
   - Proteins are the most abundant buffers in the body, especially in the intracellular fluid and plasma.
   - Hemoglobin in red blood cells is a significant buffer, binding to hydrogen ions and helping to maintain pH in blood.
   - Proteins have side chains that can either accept or donate hydrogen ions. In acidic conditions, amine groups (NH2) bind H+ to become NH3+, and in alkaline conditions, carboxyl groups (COOH) release H+ to become COO-.

## Role of Buffer Systems in Daily Physiological Processes

The body's buffer systems are constantly at work, neutralizing pH variations that result from:

- Cellular metabolism: Metabolic activities produce acids such as lactic acid and carbon dioxide, which are buffered to prevent pH shifts.
- Dietary influences: Foods that metabolize into acids or bases can alter blood pH, countered by buffer systems.
- Exercise: During intense exercise, lactic acid levels rise, necessitating immediate buffering to prevent acidosis.

## Importance of Buffer Systems in Health

The efficiency of buffer systems is crucial for health. Disruption in these systems can lead to conditions such as:

- **Acidosis**: When the body's fluids contain too much acid, leading to decreased pH.
- **Alkalosis**: When the body's fluids have excess base, leading to increased pH.
- Both conditions can disturb cellular activities and metabolic functions.

## Conclusion

The buffer systems in the human body are vital in maintaining the pH within a range compatible with life. They exemplify the body's remarkable capacity for homeostasis, seamlessly responding to and correcting deviations in pH. These systems are fundamental to our understanding of physiological processes and the impact of external factors like diet and lifestyle on our body's internal environment. The following chapters will further explore how dietary choices influence these buffer systems and overall pH balance.

## Chapter 2: Impact of Diet on Body pH

## Long-term Effects of Acidic Diets

## Potential Health Risks of pH Imbalances

The human body's pH balance is a critical factor in overall health, influencing various physiological processes. While the body is equipped with robust mechanisms to maintain this balance, certain lifestyle choices and health conditions can lead to pH imbalances. This chapter explores the potential health risks associated with both acidic and alkaline imbalances in the body.

## Health Risks of Acidic pH Imbalances

An overly acidic internal environment, or acidosis, can arise from dietary habits, chronic diseases, or other lifestyle factors. It can lead to several health issues:

1. **Osteoporosis**:
   - Chronic acidosis can lead to the leaching of calcium from bones to neutralize excess acid, potentially weakening bones and increasing the risk of osteoporosis.
   - Studies have shown a correlation between a diet high in acid-forming foods and decreased bone density.
2. **Muscle Wasting**:
   - In an acidic environment, the body may break down muscle tissue to free up amino acids that can help neutralize acidity.
   - This process can lead to muscle wasting, especially in older adults or individuals with chronic diseases.
3. **Kidney Stones**:
   - Acidosis can increase the risk of forming certain types of kidney stones. Acidic urine can lead to the crystallization of calcium and uric acid, forming stones.
   - Dietary factors, like high consumption of animal proteins, can contribute to this risk.
4. **Cardiovascular Stress**:
   - Acidosis can cause inflammation and stress on the cardiovascular system, potentially leading to an increased risk of heart disease.
   - The relationship between dietary acid load and cardiovascular health is an area of ongoing research.

## Health Risks of Alkaline pH Imbalances

Alkalosis, a condition where the body is too alkaline, is less common but can also pose health risks:

1. **Electrolyte Imbalance**:
   - Alkalosis can lead to an imbalance in electrolytes, crucial for nerve and muscle function.
   - Symptoms can include muscle cramps, spasms, and weakness.
2. **Confusion and Seizures**:
   - Severe alkalosis can affect brain function, leading to confusion, hand tremor, light-headedness, or even seizures.
   - It can be caused by prolonged vomiting, hyperventilation, or excessive bicarbonate intake.

## Dietary Influence on pH and Potential Risks

The diet plays a significant but complex role in influencing the body's pH:

1. **High Acid-Forming Diets**:
   - Diets high in animal proteins, processed foods, and low in fruits and vegetables can contribute to a higher acid load.
   - Long-term consumption of such diets can strain the body's buffering systems, potentially leading to acidosis and associated health risks.
2. **Excessive Alkaline Diets**:
   - While less common, excessively alkaline diets or the misuse of supplements like bicarbonate can lead to alkalosis.
   - Balance is key, as both extremes can be harmful.

## Conclusion

Understanding the potential health risks associated with pH imbalances highlights the importance of maintaining a balanced diet and lifestyle. While the body's buffering systems are effective at managing pH, chronic dietary and lifestyle factors can challenge these systems. A diet rich in a variety of fruits, vegetables, whole grains, and lean proteins, coupled with regular physical activity, is essential for supporting these natural regulatory mechanisms and promoting overall health. The next chapter will delve into the benefits of an alkaline diet and how it can help in mitigating these risks.

**Case Studies and Research on pH Balance and Health**

The impact of pH balance on health has been the subject of numerous studies and research. This chapter delves into a selection of case studies and research findings that illuminate the complex relationship between dietary choices, pH balance, and overall health outcomes.

**1. Research on Diet and Bone Health**

A significant area of research has focused on the connection between dietary acid load and bone health. One landmark study observed the dietary habits and bone mineral density of a large cohort over several years:

- **Findings**: Researchers found that diets high in acid-forming foods (mainly animal proteins) were associated with lower bone density.
- **Interpretation**: This was attributed to the body using calcium, a base, from bones to neutralize excess acid.
- **Counterarguments**: However, other studies argue that protein intake is beneficial for bone health due to its role in bone formation and maintenance.

**2. Studies on Kidney Stones**

The formation of kidney stones in relation to diet and body pH has been another focal point:

- **Case Study**: Patients with a history of kidney stones were observed under different dietary conditions.
- **Results**: Diets high in animal proteins, which increase acid load, were linked to a higher incidence of certain types of kidney stones.
- **Mechanism**: The acidity was found to increase calcium and oxalate concentrations in urine, key components in kidney stone formation.

**3. Acidosis and Muscle Wasting**

Research has also explored the effects of acidosis on muscle mass, particularly in older populations:

- **Study Design**: Older adults were studied for muscle mass and dietary habits.
- **Outcome**: A correlation was found between a high dietary acid load and reduced muscle mass.
- **Explanation**: The proposed mechanism is the body's use of amino acids from muscles to combat acidity.

## 4. Dietary Acid Load and Cardiovascular Risk

Emerging research suggests a link between dietary acid load and cardiovascular health:

- **Observational Studies**: These studies have shown a possible association between high dietary acid load and increased risk factors for cardiovascular disease.
- **Challenges**: Establishing a direct causal relationship remains challenging due to the complexity of dietary patterns and lifestyle factors.

## 5. Alkaline Diets and Cancer Treatment

The idea that an alkaline diet can influence cancer treatment has garnered attention:

- **Research Overview**: Some laboratory studies have suggested that cancer cells thrive in acidic environments.
- **Clinical Evidence**: However, clinical evidence supporting the effectiveness of alkaline diets in cancer treatment is limited.
- **Current Consensus**: Most health experts agree that while a balanced diet is crucial for cancer patients, altering body pH is not a viable cancer treatment strategy.

## 6. Alkaline Water and Health Benefits

The consumption of alkaline water has been touted for various health benefits:

- **Study Findings**: Some studies suggest alkaline water may help with acid reflux by denaturing pepsin.
- **Broader Research**: However, broader research on its benefits is still limited and inconclusive.

## Conclusion

These case studies and research findings highlight the intricate relationship between diet, pH balance, and health. They underscore the importance of a nuanced approach to dietary choices and the need for further research in this area. Understanding the complexities of pH balance and health can inform better dietary and lifestyle decisions, contributing to improved overall well-being. The subsequent chapters will explore practical ways to balance dietary pH and the role of specific foods and diets in maintaining optimal health.

**Benefits of an Alkaline Diet**

**Preventive health benefits**

The concept of maintaining a balanced pH in the body is not just about avoiding negative health outcomes; it also plays a significant role in preventive health. A diet that helps maintain a good acid-base balance can contribute to overall well-being and prevent various health issues. This chapter explores the preventive health benefits associated with a balanced pH diet.

**1. Enhanced Bone Health**

One of the most significant preventive benefits of maintaining a balanced pH is the positive impact on bone health.

- **Mechanism**: A diet rich in alkaline foods, particularly fruits and vegetables, can reduce calcium excretion and decrease the risk of osteoporosis.
- **Research**: Studies have shown that higher fruit and vegetable intake is associated with greater bone mineral density and reduced bone loss over time.

**2. Improved Muscle Function**

The maintenance of muscle mass and function is another area where pH balance plays a critical role, especially in aging populations.

- **Benefits**: An alkaline-leaning diet can help in preserving muscle mass and strength.
- **Studies**: Research indicates that diets lower in acid-forming foods and higher in alkaline-forming foods are associated with better muscle performance and less muscle wasting.

**3. Kidney Health**

The kidneys are directly involved in regulating the body's acid-base balance, and a balanced pH diet can support kidney health.

- **Prevention**: Diets with a balanced pH may reduce the risk of forming kidney stones and help in managing chronic kidney disease.
- **Evidence**: Clinical studies suggest that an alkaline diet may help to reduce the strain on kidneys by decreasing acid load.

## 4. Cardiovascular Benefits

The relationship between dietary pH balance and cardiovascular health is an area of growing research interest.

- **Potential Effects**: A balanced pH diet, rich in fruits, vegetables, and whole grains, has been linked to lower blood pressure and a reduced risk of hypertension and stroke.
- **Mechanism**: This effect is partly attributed to the dietary fiber, antioxidants, and phytochemicals present in these foods.

## 5. Digestive Health

The body's digestive system also benefits from a balanced pH, particularly in terms of gut health and the prevention of gastroesophageal reflux disease (GERD).

- **Alkaline Foods**: Foods such as vegetables, fruits, and nuts that are alkaline-forming can promote healthy gut flora and provide relief from acid reflux symptoms.
- **Research**: Studies have found that a diet high in acidic foods can exacerbate GERD symptoms, whereas an alkaline diet can provide symptomatic relief.

## 6. General Well-being and Chronic Disease Prevention

A diet that promotes a balanced pH is generally rich in essential nutrients, which contribute to overall health and the prevention of chronic diseases.

- **Nutritional Benefits**: Alkaline diets are typically high in vitamins, minerals, and antioxidants, which are crucial for maintaining health and preventing diseases like diabetes, hypertension, and certain cancers.
- **Lifestyle Factor**: Adopting a diet that promotes pH balance often goes hand-in-hand with other healthy lifestyle choices, further enhancing overall health.

## Conclusion

The preventive health benefits of maintaining a balanced pH through diet are multifaceted and significant. By focusing on a diet rich in alkaline-forming foods, particularly fruits and vegetables, while moderating the intake of acid-forming foods, individuals can support their bone health, muscle function, kidney health, cardiovascular health, and digestive wellness. This holistic approach to diet and health not only helps in preventing specific health issues but also contributes to overall well-being and longevity. The following chapters will delve deeper into how to incorporate a pH-balanced diet into daily life and the specific roles of various foods in achieving this balance.

**Improving Overall Wellness through pH Balance**

The pursuit of overall wellness is multifaceted, involving nutrition, physical activity, mental health, and more. Among these factors, maintaining a balanced pH through diet and lifestyle choices can play a significant role. This chapter discusses how a pH-balanced approach to living can contribute to improving overall wellness.

**1. Nutritional Balance and Diet Quality**

A pH-balanced diet typically emphasizes the consumption of fruits, vegetables, whole grains, and lean proteins, while limiting processed and high-sugar foods.

- **Broad Spectrum of Nutrients**: This dietary approach ensures a rich intake of essential vitamins, minerals, antioxidants, and dietary fiber, contributing to overall nutritional quality.
- **Preventive Nutrition**: Such a diet can prevent nutrient deficiencies and chronic conditions like obesity, heart disease, and type 2 diabetes.

**2. Enhanced Digestive Health**

The digestive system benefits significantly from a diet that maintains a balanced pH.

- **Gut Health**: Alkaline-forming foods like fruits and vegetables promote a healthy gut microbiome, improving digestion and absorption of nutrients.
- **Reduced Acid Reflux**: A balanced diet can also alleviate symptoms of acid reflux and GERD, contributing to digestive comfort and health.

**3. Bone Strength and Muscle Function**

Maintaining a balanced pH is essential for bone health and muscle function, especially as we age.

- **Bone Density**: A diet rich in alkaline-forming minerals like calcium, potassium, and magnesium supports bone density and may reduce the risk of osteoporosis.
- **Muscle Preservation**: Adequate protein intake, along with a balance of alkaline foods, helps in maintaining muscle mass and strength.

**4. Kidney Function and Detoxification**

The kidneys play a crucial role in maintaining pH balance and overall detoxification.

- **Reduced Kidney Stress**: A balanced diet supports kidney function by preventing excessive acidity, which can strain these organs.
- **Enhanced Detoxification**: Adequate hydration and consumption of nutrient-rich foods aid in the natural detoxification processes of the body.

## 5. Cardiovascular Health

The heart and vascular system also benefit from a diet that supports pH balance.

- **Blood Pressure Regulation**: Diets rich in fruits, vegetables, and low in processed foods can help manage blood pressure.
- **Reduced Inflammation**: Many alkaline-forming foods have anti-inflammatory properties, which are beneficial for cardiovascular health.

## 6. Weight Management and Metabolic Health

A balanced pH diet is often naturally lower in calories and higher in fiber, aiding in weight management.

- **Healthy Weight Loss**: Such a diet promotes a healthy and sustainable approach to weight loss.
- **Improved Metabolic Markers**: It can also improve insulin sensitivity and other metabolic markers.

## 7. Mental Well-being and Cognitive Function

Diet can impact not just physical health but also mental well-being and cognitive function.

- **Mood Enhancement**: Nutrient-rich diets have been linked to improved mood and reduced risk of depression.
- **Cognitive Health**: Diets high in antioxidants and anti-inflammatory compounds may protect against cognitive decline.

## 8. Holistic Approach to Lifestyle

Adopting a pH-balanced diet often encourages a more holistic approach to health, including regular physical activity, adequate sleep, and stress management.

- **Physical Activity**: Regular exercise complements the benefits of a balanced diet.
- **Sleep and Stress**: Quality sleep and effective stress management are integral to overall wellness.

## Conclusion

Improving overall wellness through pH balance is about more than just food choices; it's a comprehensive lifestyle approach. By focusing on a diet rich in whole, nutrient-dense foods and adopting healthy lifestyle habits, individuals can significantly enhance their physical, mental, and emotional well-being.

## Chapter 3: Evaluating and Balancing Your Diet

### Measuring the pH of Foods
### Tools and techniques

Achieving and maintaining an optimal pH balance involves a combination of monitoring techniques and dietary planning tools. This chapter provides specific tools and techniques, outlined in bullet points, to assist in managing dietary pH and ensuring a balanced intake of acidic and alkaline foods.

### Monitoring Tools

1. **pH Testing Strips:**
   - Used for testing the pH of saliva or urine.
   - Provide a quick and easy way to monitor the body's acid-alkaline balance.
   - Ideal to use first thing in the morning or two hours after eating.
2. **Digital pH Meters:**
   - Offer a more precise measurement than strips.
   - Can be used for saliva, urine, or even testing the pH of water and foods.
3. **Food pH Charts:**
   - Lists of foods categorized by their acid or alkaline-forming potential.
   - Useful for meal planning and grocery shopping.
4. **Dietary Journaling Apps:**
   - Track food and beverage intake.
   - Some apps offer insights into the acid-alkaline content of various foods.

## Dietary Planning Techniques

1. **Creating Balanced Meal Plans**:
   - Aim for a ratio that supports your pH goals, like 70% alkaline-forming foods and 30% acid-forming foods.
   - Include a variety of fruits, vegetables, whole grains, lean proteins, and healthy fats.
2. **Alkaline and Acidic Food Pairing**:
   - Combine acidic and alkaline foods in meals to create balance.
   - Example: Pair a piece of grilled chicken (acidic) with a large salad (alkaline).
3. **Portion Control**:
   - Moderate the portions of acid-forming foods like meat and cheese.
   - Increase the portions of alkaline-forming foods like vegetables and fruits.
4. **Incorporating Alkaline Superfoods**:
   - Regularly include high-alkaline foods like kale, spinach, cucumber, avocado, and almonds.
5. **Cooking Methods**:
   - Opt for steaming, grilling, or roasting rather than frying.
   - Cooking with less oil and more herbs and spices to enhance the alkalinity of meals.

## Techniques for Food and Beverage Choices

1. **Hydration with pH in Mind**:
   - Drink plenty of water throughout the day.
   - Consider alkaline water or adding lemon to water for an alkalizing effect.
2. **Mindful Snacking**:
   - Choose snacks that are high in alkalinity, like raw nuts, seeds, or fresh fruit.
   - Avoid processed snacks that are typically high in acid-forming ingredients.
3. **Limiting Acid-Forming Beverages**:
   - Reduce intake of coffee, alcohol, and sugary drinks.
   - Replace with herbal teas, green tea, or vegetable juices.

## Supplementation and pH Balance

1. **Alkaline Mineral Supplements**:
   - In certain cases, supplements like potassium or magnesium can help in maintaining alkalinity.
   - Consult with a healthcare provider before starting any supplements.
2. **Probiotics and Digestive Enzymes**:
   - Aid in digestion and can indirectly support pH balance.
   - Probiotics are beneficial for gut health, which is important for overall pH regulation.

## Conclusion

Monitoring and managing dietary pH through these specific tools and techniques can significantly contribute to achieving a balanced pH diet. By incorporating these strategies into daily routines, individuals can actively work towards enhancing their overall health and wellness. The subsequent chapters will focus on specific alkaline food recipes, diet plans, and transitioning tips to an alkaline diet for improved health.

**pH values of common foods**

Understanding the pH values of common foods can greatly assist in managing a balanced diet. This chapter lists various foods, categorized by their general pH levels and their impact on the body's pH balance. It's important to note that the pH value of food does not directly correspond to its effect on the body's pH; rather, it is the ash residue after digestion that determines whether a food is acidifying or alkalizing.

## Highly Acidic Foods (pH 0-4.5)

These foods have a low pH and are generally considered acidic. However, some may have an alkalizing effect after digestion.

- **Citrus Fruits**:
    - Lemons (pH 2-3)
    - Limes (pH 2-2.8)
    - Oranges (pH 3-4)
- **Berries**:
    - Strawberries (pH 3-3.5)
    - Blueberries (pH 3-3.2)
- **Vinegar-Based Products**:
    - Apple Cider Vinegar (pH 2.5-3)
    - White Vinegar (pH 2.4)
- **Fermented Foods**:
    - Sauerkraut (pH 3.1-3.6)
    - Yogurt (pH 3.5-4.5)

## Moderately Acidic Foods (pH 4.6-5.5)

These foods are slightly less acidic and include certain dairy products and grains.

- **Dairy Products**:
    - Cow's Milk (pH 4.6-4.8)
    - Cheese (pH varies widely, generally around 5)
- **Grains**:
    - White Bread (pH 5-5.5)
    - Whole Wheat Bread (pH 5.5)

## Neutral Foods (pH 6-7)

These foods are close to neutral in pH and include fats and oils.

- **Fats and Oils**:
    - Olive Oil (pH 7)
    - Butter (pH 6.1-6.4)

## Mildly Alkaline Foods (pH 7.1-8)

These foods are slightly alkaline. Most of them are fruits and vegetables.

- **Vegetables**:
    - Spinach (pH 7.2-7.5)
    - Cucumbers (pH 7.1-7.6)
- **Fruits**:
    - Bananas (pH 7.1-7.5)
    - Avocados (pH 7.5-7.8)

## Highly Alkaline Foods (pH 8.1-9)

These foods are very alkaline and great for balancing an acidic diet.

- **Leafy Greens**:
    - Kale (pH 8.5)
    - Swiss Chard (pH 8.3)
- **Root Vegetables**:
    - Carrots (pH 8.1-8.3)
    - Beets (pH 8.2-8.5)

## Special Mention: Alkalizing vs. Acidifying Effects

- **Citrus Fruits**:
    - Despite their low pH, they have an alkalizing effect on the body due to their mineral content.
- **Dairy Products**:
    - Generally acid-forming due to their high protein and phosphorus content.

## Conclusion

This chapter provides a basic guide to the pH values of common foods and their potential impact on the body's pH balance. It's important to balance the intake of acidic and alkaline foods to maintain good health. The next chapter will delve into creating a balanced diet, which incorporates these foods in appropriate proportions for optimal health and well-being.

**Creating a Balanced Diet**

**Proportions of acidic vs alkaline foods**

Creating a balanced diet that supports your body's pH involves understanding the right proportions of acidic and alkaline foods. This chapter outlines specific guidelines and proportions to help you achieve a harmonious dietary balance.

**Understanding the Ideal Balance**

The goal is not to eliminate acidic foods but to strike a balance with alkaline foods. A commonly recommended ratio for general health is approximately:

- **60-80% Alkaline-Forming Foods**: Fruits, vegetables, nuts, and seeds.
- **20-40% Acid-Forming Foods**: Grains, meats, dairy products, and processed foods.

**Specific Guidelines**

1. **Daily Fruit and Vegetable Intake**:
    - Aim for at least 5 servings of vegetables and 2-3 servings of fruits daily.
    - Include leafy greens and a variety of colorful vegetables.
2. **Moderation of Animal Proteins**:
    - Limit red meat and pork to 1-2 times per week.
    - Opt for lean proteins like chicken, turkey, or fish.
    - Incorporate plant-based proteins like beans and lentils.
3. **Dairy and Alternative Choices**:
    - If consuming dairy, opt for low-fat options in moderation.
    - Consider plant-based alternatives like almond milk or coconut yogurt.
4. **Selecting Grains**:
    - Choose whole grains over processed ones (e.g., brown rice over white rice).
    - Limit intake of bread, especially white bread, and processed cereals.
5. **Incorporating Nuts and Seeds**:
    - Add a handful of almonds, chia seeds, or flaxseeds to your daily diet.
    - Use nuts and seeds as snacks or toppings for salads and yogurt.
6. **Hydration**:
    - Drink at least 8-10 glasses of water daily.
    - Herbal teas and lemon water are good alkaline options.
7. **Limiting Processed Foods and Sugars**:
    - Avoid excessive consumption of processed foods, sugary snacks, and beverages.

## Balancing Meals with Acidic and Alkaline Foods

1. **Breakfast**:
   - Alkaline: Fresh fruit or a smoothie with spinach, avocado, and almond milk.
   - Acidic: If adding yogurt or eggs, balance with a side of alkaline fruits or vegetables.
2. **Lunch and Dinner**:
   - Alkaline: A large portion of your plate should be vegetables, either raw, steamed, or lightly cooked.
   - Acidic: Accompany with a smaller portion of protein or grain.
3. **Snacks**:
   - Alkaline: Fresh fruits, vegetables, or a small portion of nuts.
   - Acidic: Cheese or yogurt in moderation, balanced with alkaline fruits.

## Meal Planning Tips

- **Variety is Key**: Ensure a wide range of fruits, vegetables, grains, and proteins.
- **Portion Control**: Be mindful of portion sizes, especially for acid-forming foods.
- **Cooking Methods**: Favor steaming, grilling, or sautéing over frying.
- **Seasonal and Local Foods**: Opt for fresh, in-season produce for higher alkalinity.

## Conclusion

Balancing the proportions of acidic and alkaline foods in your diet is crucial for maintaining optimal health and supporting your body's natural pH balance. By following these specific guidelines and adjusting portions accordingly, you can create a diet that not only tastes good but also nourishes your body effectively. The next chapters will provide detailed recipes and meal plans to help you incorporate these principles into your everyday eating habits.

**Incorporating variety and nutrition**

A key aspect of a pH-balanced diet is not just focusing on the acid-alkaline spectrum but also ensuring that the diet is varied and nutritionally complete. This chapter outlines strategies to incorporate both variety and essential nutrients into your diet, ensuring it is balanced, enjoyable, and beneficial for overall health.

## 1. Emphasizing Nutrient-Dense Foods

- **Whole Foods Over Processed**: Choose whole fruits, vegetables, whole grains, and lean proteins over processed foods.
- **Colorful Vegetables and Fruits**: Include a rainbow of fruits and vegetables to ensure a wide range of vitamins, minerals, and antioxidants.
- **Healthy Fats**: Incorporate sources of good fats such as avocados, nuts, seeds, and olive oil.

## 2. Diverse Protein Sources

- **Plant-Based Proteins**: Add variety with plant-based proteins like beans, lentils, chickpeas, tofu, and tempeh.
- **Lean Animal Proteins**: Opt for lean cuts of meat, fish, and poultry. Include fish at least twice a week for omega-3 fatty acids.
- **Dairy and Alternatives**: Choose low-fat dairy products or plant-based alternatives like almond, soy, or oat milk.

## 3. Whole Grains and Fiber

- **Whole Grains**: Select whole grains like quinoa, brown rice, barley, and whole wheat, which are higher in nutrients and fiber compared to refined grains.
- **High-Fiber Foods**: Increase intake of high-fiber foods like beans, legumes, fruits, and vegetables to support digestive health.

## 4. Healthy Fats

- **Sources of Omega-3s**: Incorporate fatty fish like salmon, mackerel, and sardines, and plant sources like flaxseeds and walnuts.
- **Cooking Oils**: Use healthier oils like olive oil and avocado oil for cooking and dressings.

## 5. Hydration

- **Water Intake**: Aim for 8-10 glasses of water per day, more if you are active or live in a hot climate.
- **Herbal Teas**: Herbal teas can be a hydrating, alkaline-forming beverage option.
- **Limiting Caffeine and Alcohol**: Reduce intake of caffeine and alcoholic beverages, which can be dehydrating and acid-forming.

## 6. Balancing Micronutrients

- **Vitamins and Minerals**: Ensure a diet rich in essential vitamins and minerals by consuming a variety of fruits, vegetables, nuts, seeds, and lean proteins.
- **Supplements**: Consider supplements if you have specific dietary restrictions or deficiencies, but consult a healthcare professional first.

## 7. Seasonal and Local Foods

- **Seasonal Eating**: Choose seasonal produce for better flavor, nutritional value, and environmental sustainability.
- **Local Produce**: Buying local supports the community and often provides fresher, more nutrient-rich foods.

## 8. Experimenting with International Cuisines

- **Cultural Diversity**: Experiment with recipes from different cultures to add variety to your diet.
- **Spices and Herbs**: Use a variety of spices and herbs not only for flavor but also for their health benefits.

## 9. Mindful Eating

- **Listening to Your Body**: Pay attention to how different foods make you feel and adjust your diet accordingly.
- **Enjoying Meals**: Take time to savor and enjoy your meals, which can aid in digestion and satisfaction.

## 10. Regular Meal Planning

- **Planning Ahead**: Plan meals weekly to ensure a balanced diet and prevent last-minute unhealthy choices.
- **Prepping in Advance**: Meal prep can save time and make it easier to eat healthily.

## Conclusion

Incorporating variety and nutrition into a pH-balanced diet is about more than just managing acidity and alkalinity; it's about creating a holistic approach to eating that is enjoyable, sustainable, and health-promoting. By embracing a diverse range of nutrient-dense foods and mindful eating practices, you can enjoy the full spectrum of flavors and benefits that a balanced diet offers. The upcoming chapters will provide practical meal ideas and recipes to help integrate these principles into everyday life.

## Chapter 4: Alkaline Food Recipes and Diet Plans

### Delicious Alkaline Recipes

### Breakfast, lunch, dinner, and snacks

### Breakfast Recipes

1. **Spinach and Mushroom Omelette**
   - Ingredients: 2 eggs, 1 cup spinach, ½ cup mushrooms, 1 tbsp olive oil, salt, pepper, ¼ cup grated cheese (optional).
   - Instructions: Sauté spinach and mushrooms in olive oil. Beat eggs and pour over the veggies in a pan. Cook until set, flip, add cheese, fold, and serve.
2. **Almond Butter and Banana Oatmeal**
   - Ingredients: ½ cup rolled oats, 1 cup almond milk, 1 banana, 1 tbsp almond butter, cinnamon.
   - Instructions: Cook oats in almond milk, stirring occasionally. Slice banana on top, add a dollop of almond butter, and sprinkle with cinnamon.
3. **Avocado Toast with Poached Egg**
   - Ingredients: 1 slice whole grain bread, 1 avocado, 1 egg, lemon juice, salt, pepper.
   - Instructions: Toast bread, mash avocado with lemon juice, salt, and pepper. Spread on toast. Top with a poached egg.
4. **Berry Smoothie Bowl**
   - Ingredients: 1 cup mixed berries, 1 banana, ½ cup Greek yogurt, 1 tbsp honey, toppings (chia seeds, granola, sliced almonds).
   - Instructions: Blend berries, banana, yogurt, and honey until smooth. Pour into a bowl and add desired toppings.

**Lunch Recipes**

1. **Quinoa and Black Bean Salad**
   - Ingredients: 1 cup cooked quinoa, ½ cup black beans, 1 diced tomato, ½ diced cucumber, 1 diced avocado, lime juice, olive oil, salt, cilantro.
   - Instructions: Mix all ingredients in a bowl, dress with lime juice, olive oil, and salt. Garnish with cilantro.
2. **Grilled Chicken and Kale Salad**
   - Ingredients: 1 grilled chicken breast, 2 cups kale, ½ cup sliced strawberries, ¼ cup feta cheese, balsamic vinaigrette.
   - Instructions: Toss kale, strawberries, and feta. Top with sliced grilled chicken and drizzle with vinaigrette.
3. **Vegetable Stir-Fry with Tofu**
   - Ingredients: 1 cup mixed vegetables (broccoli, bell peppers, carrots), ½ block tofu, 2 tbsp soy sauce, 1 tbsp sesame oil, garlic, ginger.
   - Instructions: Stir-fry tofu until golden. Add vegetables, garlic, ginger, and stir-fry until cooked. Add soy sauce and sesame oil.
4. **Tomato and Basil Pasta**
   - Ingredients: 2 cups whole wheat pasta, 1 cup cherry tomatoes, fresh basil, 2 cloves garlic, olive oil, parmesan cheese.
   - Instructions: Cook pasta, sauté tomatoes and garlic in olive oil. Combine with pasta, add basil and top with parmesan.

## Dinner Recipes

1. **Baked Salmon with Asparagus**
   - o Ingredients: 2 salmon fillets, 1 bunch asparagus, lemon slices, olive oil, salt, pepper, dill.
   - o Instructions: Place salmon and asparagus on a baking sheet. Drizzle with olive oil, season, top with lemon and dill. Bake at 400°F for 20 mins.
2. **Lentil Soup**
   - o Ingredients: 1 cup lentils, 1 onion, 2 carrots, 2 celery stalks, vegetable broth, 1 can diced tomatoes, thyme, salt, pepper.
   - o Instructions: Sauté onion, carrots, and celery. Add lentils, broth, tomatoes, and thyme. Simmer until lentils are tender. Season to taste.
3. **Stuffed Bell Peppers**
   - o Ingredients: 4 bell peppers, 1 cup brown rice, 1 cup black beans, corn, diced tomatoes, cumin, cheese.
   - o Instructions: Mix cooked rice, beans, corn, tomatoes, and cumin. Stuff into bell peppers, top with cheese, bake at 375°F for 30 mins.
4. **Beef and Broccoli Stir-Fry**
   - o Ingredients: Sliced beef, 2 cups broccoli, soy sauce, garlic, ginger, olive oil, cornstarch, beef broth.
   - o Instructions: Stir-fry beef, set aside. Stir-fry broccoli with garlic and ginger. Add beef, sauce (soy sauce, broth, cornstarch), cook until thickened.

## Snack Recipes

1. **Greek Yogurt with Honey and Walnuts**
   - o Ingredients: 1 cup Greek yogurt, 2 tbsp honey, a handful of walnuts.
   - o Instructions: Mix yogurt with honey, top with walnuts.
2. **Hummus and Veggie Sticks**
   - o Ingredients: Hummus, sliced carrots, cucumbers, bell peppers.
   - o Instructions: Serve hummus with sliced vegetables for dipping.
3. **Apple Slices with Almond Butter**
   - o Ingredients: 1 apple, almond butter.
   - o Instructions: Slice apple and serve with a side of almond butter.
4. **Oatmeal and Raisin Energy Balls**
   - o Ingredients: 1 cup rolled oats, ½ cup almond butter, ¼ cup honey, ½ cup raisins.
   - o Instructions: Mix ingredients, roll into balls, refrigerate until set.

## 3-Ingredient Recipes for Each Meal of the Day

## Breakfast

1. **Banana Pancakes**
   - Ingredients: 2 ripe bananas, 2 eggs, ½ cup of oat flour.
   - Instructions: Mash bananas, whisk in eggs, and stir in oat flour to form a batter. Cook on a non-stick skillet over medium heat until golden brown on each side.
2. **Yogurt Parfait**
   - Ingredients: Greek yogurt, mixed berries, granola.
   - Instructions: Layer Greek yogurt, mixed berries, and granola in a glass or bowl. Repeat layers until ingredients are used up.
3. **Avocado Toast**
   - Ingredients: 1 avocado, 2 slices of whole grain bread, salt.
   - Instructions: Toast bread, mash avocado with a pinch of salt, and spread over the toast.

## Lunch

1. **Caprese Salad**
   - Ingredients: Sliced tomatoes, fresh mozzarella cheese, fresh basil leaves.
   - Instructions: Layer slices of tomato and mozzarella cheese alternately on a plate, garnish with basil leaves.
2. **Turkey Roll-Ups**
   - Ingredients: Sliced turkey breast, cream cheese, cucumber strips.
   - Instructions: Spread cream cheese on turkey slices, place a cucumber strip on each, and roll them up.
3. **Chickpea Salad**
   - Ingredients: Canned chickpeas, diced cucumber, Italian dressing.
   - Instructions: Mix chickpeas and cucumber, drizzle with Italian dressing, and toss to coat.

## Dinner

1. **Pesto Pasta**
   - Ingredients: Pasta, pesto sauce, grated Parmesan cheese.
   - Instructions: Cook pasta according to package instructions, drain, mix with pesto sauce, and top with Parmesan cheese.
2. **Baked Chicken Thighs**
   - Ingredients: Chicken thighs, olive oil, your favorite seasoning blend.
   - Instructions: Coat chicken thighs in olive oil and seasoning, bake at 375°F for 35-40 minutes or until fully cooked.
3. **Stir-Fried Tofu and Broccoli**
   - Ingredients: Firm tofu, broccoli florets, soy sauce.
   - Instructions: Pan-fry tofu until golden, add broccoli, and stir-fry until tender. Drizzle with soy sauce and cook for another minute.

## Snacks

1. **Fruit Skewers**
   - Ingredients: Strawberries, grapes, and pineapple chunks.
   - Instructions: Thread strawberries, grapes, and pineapple chunks onto skewers.
2. **Peanut Butter Celery Sticks**
   - Ingredients: Celery sticks, peanut butter, raisins.
   - Instructions: Fill celery sticks with peanut butter and top with raisins.
3. **Almond-Stuffed Dates**
   - Ingredients: Pitted dates, almonds, dark chocolate chips.
   - Instructions: Insert an almond into each date, then top with a dark chocolate chip.

## Sample Diet Plans

## Weekly meal planning

Weekly meal planning is a strategic approach to eating that not only ensures a balanced pH diet but also saves time, reduces stress, and helps in maintaining healthy eating habits. This chapter outlines a systematic approach to meal planning, focusing on incorporating a variety of acidic and alkaline foods throughout the week.

### Understanding the Basics of Meal Planning

1. **Assess Dietary Needs**: Consider your health goals, dietary preferences, and any specific nutritional requirements.
2. **Balance of Acidic and Alkaline Foods**: Aim for a mix of about 60-80% alkaline-forming foods and 20-40% acid-forming foods in your weekly plan.
3. **Portion Control**: Be mindful of serving sizes, especially for acid-forming foods like meats and dairy.

### Steps for Effective Meal Planning

1. **Create a Menu for the Week**:
   - Plan for all meals – breakfast, lunch, dinner, and snacks.
   - Incorporate a variety of foods to ensure nutritional balance and prevent monotony.
2. **Draft a Grocery List**:
   - Based on your menu, list all ingredients needed.
   - Organize the list by store sections (produce, dairy, meats, pantry items) for efficiency.
3. **Shop Wisely**:
   - Stick to your list to avoid impulse buys.
   - Opt for fresh, whole foods and minimize processed items.
4. **Prep in Advance**:
   - Dedicate time to food prep after shopping.
   - Wash and chop vegetables, cook grains, marinate proteins, and portion out snacks.
5. **Flexible and Practical Approach**:
   - Be realistic about the time you have for cooking.
   - Incorporate simple and quick recipes for busy days.

## Sample Weekly Meal Plan

*Note: This plan assumes a mix of alkaline and acidic foods for a balanced pH diet.*

### Monday

- Breakfast: Greek yogurt with honey and walnuts.
- Lunch: Quinoa and black bean salad.
- Dinner: Grilled chicken with steamed broccoli and brown rice.
- Snacks: Hummus with carrot sticks.

### Tuesday

- Breakfast: Oatmeal with sliced bananas and almond butter.
- Lunch: Turkey and avocado wrap with whole-grain tortilla.
- Dinner: Baked salmon with a side salad (leafy greens, cucumber, cherry tomatoes).
- Snacks: Fresh fruit salad.

### Wednesday

- Breakfast: Smoothie with spinach, banana, and almond milk.
- Lunch: Lentil soup with a side of whole-grain bread.
- Dinner: Stir-fried tofu and mixed vegetables over quinoa.
- Snacks: Celery sticks with peanut butter.

### Thursday

- Breakfast: Scrambled eggs with sautéed mushrooms and spinach.
- Lunch: Chicken Caesar salad with light dressing.
- Dinner: Whole wheat pasta with pesto and a side of grilled vegetables.
- Snacks: Apple slices with a handful of almonds.

### Friday

- Breakfast: Avocado toast with poached egg.
- Lunch: Sushi rolls with brown rice and a seaweed salad.
- Dinner: Homemade pizza with a whole wheat base, topped with veggies and low-fat cheese.
- Snacks: Greek yogurt with mixed berries.

## Saturday

- Breakfast: Blueberry pancakes with maple syrup.
- Lunch: Grilled vegetable and hummus sandwich.
- Dinner: Beef stir-fry with bell peppers and broccoli.
- Snacks: Mixed nuts.

## Sunday

- Breakfast: Berry parfait with granola.
- Lunch: Caprese salad with fresh mozzarella, tomatoes, and basil.
- Dinner: Roasted chicken with sweet potatoes and green beans.
- Snacks: Dark chocolate and strawberries.

## Conclusion

Weekly meal planning for a pH-balanced diet is about thoughtful preparation and variety. By planning ahead, you can ensure that your meals are both nutritious and enjoyable, while also catering to the acidic and alkaline balance crucial for health. Remember, flexibility is key; adjust your plan as needed based on your schedule and preferences. The subsequent chapters will offer tips on transitioning to an alkaline diet and maintaining this balance in the long term.

## Shopping lists and prep tips

Efficient shopping and preparation are key components of maintaining a pH-balanced diet. This chapter provides detailed shopping lists and preparation tips, organized in bullet points, to help streamline your grocery shopping and meal prep process.

## Comprehensive Shopping List

**Vegetables** (Predominantly Alkaline)

- Leafy greens (spinach, kale, arugula)
- Root vegetables (carrots, beets, sweet potatoes)
- Cruciferous vegetables (broccoli, cauliflower, Brussels sprouts)
- Salad vegetables (cucumbers, bell peppers, lettuce)

**Fruits** (Predominantly Alkaline)

- Citrus fruits (lemons, oranges)
- Berries (strawberries, blueberries, raspberries)
- Apples, bananas, pears
- Avocados, grapes, melons

**Proteins**

- Lean meats (chicken, turkey, lean beef cuts)
- Fish and seafood
- Plant-based proteins (tofu, tempeh, legumes)
- Eggs, Greek yogurt (in moderation)

**Grains** (Moderate Acidic to Neutral)

- Whole grains (quinoa, brown rice, whole wheat pasta)
- Oatmeal, barley

**Nuts and Seeds** (Mostly Alkaline)

- Almonds, cashews, walnuts
- Chia seeds, flaxseeds, pumpkin seeds

**Dairy and Alternatives** (Moderate Acidic)

- Low-fat milk, cheese (in moderation)
- Plant-based milk (almond, soy, coconut)

## Beverages

- Herbal teas
- Alkaline water, mineral water

## Condiments and Spices

- Olive oil, coconut oil
- Herbs (basil, parsley, cilantro)
- Spices (turmeric, ginger, cinnamon)
- Apple cider vinegar, balsamic vinegar

## Preparation Tips

### 1. Organizing Your Grocery Shopping

- Sort your list by department (produce, dairy, meat, etc.) for efficiency.
- Shop for fresh produce twice a week to ensure freshness.
- Check for seasonal produce for better quality and pricing.

### 2. Prepping Right After Shopping

- Wash and chop vegetables for easy use during the week.
- Portion out and marinate meats and fish, then refrigerate or freeze.
- Cook grains and legumes in bulk for quick meal assembly.

### 3. Efficient Storage

- Use airtight containers to keep prepped ingredients fresh.
- Label containers with dates to track freshness.
- Store herbs in damp paper towels in the refrigerator.

### 4. Making Use of Freezer Space

- Freeze extra portions of cooked meals for busy days.
- Freeze fruits like berries for smoothies or desserts.
- Store homemade broths and sauces in ice cube trays for easy use.

### 5. Planning for Snacks

- Pre-portion nuts and seeds for grab-and-go convenience.
- Prep vegetables for snacking and store them in the fridge.
- Keep a supply of fresh fruit available for a quick, healthy option.

## 6. Simplifying Breakfast

- Overnight oats or chia seed puddings can be prepped in jars for a quick breakfast.
- Boil eggs at the start of the week for an easy protein source.

## 7. Utilizing Cooking and Baking Days

- Designate a day for more time-consuming cooking or baking.
- Prepare dishes like casseroles, soups, or healthy baked goods.

## 8. Embracing Versatility

- Mix and match prepped ingredients to create varied meals.
- Experiment with different spices and herbs to change the flavor profiles of dishes.

## Conclusion

By following these shopping and preparation tips, you can streamline the process of maintaining a pH-balanced diet. Effective planning and organization not only save time but also ensure that you have healthy, balanced meals throughout the week. The next chapter will delve into transitioning to an alkaline diet and maintaining dietary balance in the long term.

## Chapter 5: Transitioning to an Alkaline Diet

## Gradual Changes for Sustainable Health

### Tips for transitioning

Adopting a pH-balanced diet can be a significant change for many individuals. Transitioning smoothly requires understanding, patience, and a strategic approach. This chapter provides practical tips, structured in bullet points, to ease the transition to a diet that balances acidic and alkaline foods.

### Understanding the pH-Balanced Diet

- **Educate Yourself**: Learn about the principles of a pH-balanced diet, including the effects of acidic and alkaline foods on the body.
- **Set Realistic Goals**: Start with achievable goals, like incorporating more vegetables into your meals or reducing processed food intake.

### Gradual Dietary Changes

- **Introduce Alkaline Foods Slowly**: Gradually increase your intake of alkaline-forming foods like fruits and vegetables.
- **Reduce Acidic Foods Gradually**: Slowly decrease consumption of highly acidic foods, such as red meat and processed foods.
- **Experiment with Plant-Based Proteins**: Try incorporating tofu, lentils, and beans as alternatives to animal proteins.

### Meal Planning and Preparation

- **Plan Your Meals**: Create a weekly meal plan that includes a variety of alkaline and acidic foods.
- **Prep in Advance**: Prepare and store portions of alkaline foods for easy access and cooking throughout the week.
- **Cook at Home**: Cooking at home allows you to control the ingredients and the balance of your meals.

### Making Informed Food Choices

- **Read Food Labels**: Be aware of the ingredients in packaged foods to avoid high acid-forming additives.
- **Choose Whole Foods**: Focus on whole, unprocessed foods for the majority of your diet.
- **Stay Hydrated**: Drink plenty of water, herbal teas, and other hydrating, low-acid beverages.

## Lifestyle Considerations

- **Regular Exercise**: Incorporate regular physical activity, which can help the body maintain its natural pH balance.
- **Adequate Sleep**: Ensure sufficient sleep, as lack of sleep can disrupt bodily functions, including pH balance.
- **Stress Management**: Engage in stress-reducing activities, as stress can influence the body's acid levels.

## Support and Community

- **Seek Support**: Share your goals with family and friends who can offer support and accountability.
- **Join Communities**: Participate in online forums or local groups focused on pH-balanced diets for inspiration and tips.

## Adjustments Based on Feedback

- **Listen to Your Body**: Pay attention to how your body reacts to dietary changes and adjust accordingly.
- **Consult Healthcare Professionals**: Seek advice from dietitians or doctors, especially if you have health concerns or dietary restrictions.

## Exploring New Foods and Recipes

- **Try New Recipes**: Experiment with recipes that focus on alkaline ingredients.
- **Explore International Cuisines**: Many cultures incorporate a balance of acidic and alkaline foods naturally.

## Mindful Eating Habits

- **Eat Slowly**: Take time to chew your food thoroughly and enjoy your meals.
- **Mindful Choices**: Be conscious of your food choices and how they align with your pH-balance goals.

## Monitoring Progress

- **Track Your Meals**: Keep a food diary to monitor the balance of your diet.
- **Assess Your Health**: Regularly check in with how you feel physically and mentally since making the dietary changes.

## Conclusion

Transitioning to a pH-balanced diet is a journey that involves gradual changes, experimentation, and learning. By following these tips, you can make the transition smoother and more enjoyable, leading to a sustainable change in your dietary habits. The subsequent chapters will delve deeper into specific challenges you may encounter during this transition and strategies to overcome them.

## Overcoming challenges

Adopting and sustaining a pH-balanced diet can present various challenges. From dealing with cravings to managing social situations, it's important to have strategies in place. This chapter offers practical tips, organized in bullet points, to help overcome common obstacles encountered while maintaining this dietary approach.

## Dealing with Cravings

- **Understand Your Cravings**: Identify if your cravings are due to emotional eating, habit, or actual hunger.
- **Healthy Alternatives**: Find healthier alternatives that satisfy your cravings. For instance, choose dark chocolate over milk chocolate.
- **Stay Hydrated**: Sometimes thirst is mistaken for hunger. Drink water or herbal tea when a craving hits.

## Eating Out and Social Events

- **Menu Research**: Look at the menu beforehand when eating out and plan your meal choices.
- **Communicate Dietary Preferences**: Don't hesitate to communicate your dietary needs at restaurants or social gatherings.
- **Bring a Dish**: When attending a potluck or gathering, bring a pH-balanced dish you can enjoy.

## Time and Convenience

- **Meal Prepping**: Dedicate a day to meal prep for the week. This saves time and ensures you have healthy options readily available.
- **Quick and Easy Recipes**: Have a repertoire of simple, quick pH-balanced recipes for busy days.
- **Utilize Healthy Convenience Options**: Opt for healthy pre-cut vegetables, pre-cooked grains, or canned beans for quicker meal preparation.

## Budget Constraints

- **Buy in Bulk**: Purchase staples like grains, nuts, and seeds in bulk, which is often cheaper.
- **Seasonal Produce**: Buy fruits and vegetables that are in season for better prices and quality.
- **Plan Meals Around Sales**: Check local grocery flyers for sales and plan your meals accordingly.

## Family and Household Acceptance

- **Involve Family in Meal Planning**: Make meal planning a family activity, so everyone has input.
- **Educate and Share Benefits**: Share the health benefits of a pH-balanced diet with your family.
- **Introduce Changes Gradually**: Slowly incorporate more pH-balanced dishes into family meals.

## Maintaining Motivation

- **Set Realistic Goals**: Set achievable goals and celebrate when you reach them.
- **Track Progress**: Keep a food diary or journal to monitor your progress and reflect on how you feel.
- **Seek Support**: Join online communities or local groups for motivation and support.

## Navigating Misinformation

- **Educate Yourself**: Stay informed with credible sources about pH balance and nutrition.
- **Consult Health Professionals**: Seek advice from dietitians or healthcare providers for accurate information.

## Travel and Vacations

- **Plan Ahead**: Research restaurants and food options at your destination in advance.
- **Pack Snacks**: Bring pH-balanced snacks like nuts, fruits, or whole-grain bars for on-the-go.
- **Balance and Enjoy**: Choose healthier options when possible, but also allow yourself to enjoy local cuisines.

## Dealing with Setbacks

- **Be Kind to Yourself**: Understand that setbacks happen, and it's part of the journey.
- **Learn from Experiences**: Reflect on what led to the setback and how you can handle it differently in the future.
- **Get Back on Track**: Refocus on your goals and get back to your routine without guilt.

## Conclusion

Overcoming the challenges of maintaining a pH-balanced diet requires a combination of planning, flexibility, and resilience. By anticipating potential obstacles and having strategies to address them, you can successfully adhere to a diet that promotes health and well-being. The final chapter will summarize the key points of maintaining a pH-balanced diet and provide final thoughts on embarking on this nutritional journey.

## Listening to Your Body

### Identifying personal triggers

Adhering to a pH-balanced diet can be challenging, especially when personal triggers lead to dietary imbalances. Identifying and managing these triggers is crucial for maintaining a consistent and healthy eating pattern. This chapter explores various personal triggers and provides strategies to identify and manage them effectively.

### Understanding Personal Triggers

Personal triggers are specific situations, emotions, or foods that can disrupt your dietary habits. Recognizing these triggers is the first step in managing them.

### Common Dietary Triggers

- **Emotional Eating**: Turning to food for comfort during stress, sadness, or boredom.
- **Social Influences**: Overeating or choosing unhealthy options in social settings.
- **Cravings**: Strong desires for specific foods, often high in sugar, salt, or fat.
- **Habitual Eating**: Consuming certain foods out of habit, regardless of hunger.

### Strategies for Identifying Personal Triggers

1. **Keep a Food Diary**:
   - Document what you eat, when, and your emotional state at the time.
   - Review your diary to identify patterns that suggest triggers.
2. **Mindful Eating**:
   - Practice being present while eating to better understand your body's signals.
   - Notice if you're eating out of hunger or due to an external trigger.
3. **Reflect on Past Experiences**:
   - Think about times you've deviated from your diet.
   - Identify the circumstances that contributed to these instances.
4. **Pay Attention to Body Signals**:
   - Notice physical responses to certain foods or eating habits.
   - Symptoms like fatigue, digestive discomfort, or mood swings can indicate triggers.

## Managing Emotional Triggers

- **Develop Stress-Relief Techniques**: Practice relaxation methods like deep breathing, meditation, or exercise.
- **Seek Emotional Support**: Talk to friends, family, or professionals about emotional challenges.
- **Find Non-Food Coping Mechanisms**: Engage in activities like reading, walking, or hobbies to manage emotions.

## Handling Social Eating

- **Plan Ahead**: Decide what you'll eat before attending social events.
- **Bring Your Own Food**: If possible, bring a pH-balanced dish to share.
- **Practice Saying No**: Learn to politely decline food that doesn't fit your diet.

## Controlling Cravings

- **Healthy Substitutes**: Find healthier alternatives that satisfy your cravings.
- **Distraction Techniques**: Engage in an activity to distract from cravings.
- **Allow Occasional Indulgences**: Moderation is key; occasionally indulging can prevent strong cravings.

## Changing Habitual Eating

- **Alter Routines**: Change your daily routine to break habits associated with eating.
- **Substitute with Better Choices**: Replace habitual food choices with healthier options.
- **Mindful Portion Control**: Be conscious of portion sizes to avoid overeating.

## Conclusion

Identifying personal triggers is a vital aspect of maintaining a pH-balanced diet. By understanding what prompts you to deviate from your dietary goals, you can develop strategies to manage these triggers effectively. This proactive approach helps in sustaining dietary changes, contributing to long-term health and wellness. The final chapter will summarize the key principles of a pH-balanced diet and offer concluding thoughts on embracing this lifestyle for optimal health.

**Adjusting the Diet as Needed for pH Balance**

Maintaining a pH-balanced diet is not a static process; it requires continuous adjustments based on individual needs, bodily responses, and changing circumstances. This chapter outlines strategies for fine-tuning your diet to ensure it remains effective, enjoyable, and aligned with your health goals.

**Understanding the Need for Adjustments**

A one-size-fits-all approach doesn't work for dietary habits. Each individual's body responds differently to foods, and personal health goals can change over time, necessitating diet adjustments.

**1. Monitoring Body Responses**

- **Track Physical Changes**: Pay attention to changes in energy levels, digestion, skin condition, and overall well-being.
- **Assess Digestive Health**: Notice how different foods affect your digestion, identifying any that cause discomfort or irregularities.
- **Adapt to Body Signals**: If certain foods consistently cause negative reactions, consider reducing or eliminating them from your diet.

**2. Personal Health Goals**

- **Weight Management**: Adjust portions and food choices based on whether you aim to lose, gain, or maintain weight.
- **Chronic Health Conditions**: If dealing with conditions like diabetes, heart disease, or kidney problems, tailor your diet to these specific needs.

**3. Lifestyle Changes**

- **Activity Levels**: Increase nutrient-dense, energy-providing foods if your physical activity increases.
- **Age-Related Adjustments**: As you age, your nutritional needs and metabolism change, requiring dietary adjustments.

**4. Feedback from Regular Health Check-Ups**

- **Medical Advice**: Regular check-ups can provide insights into how your diet is affecting your health. Adjust based on medical advice.
- **Blood Work**: Use blood tests to assess nutrient levels and other health markers, making dietary changes as needed.

## Strategies for Adjusting Your Diet

1. **Incorporate a Wider Variety of Foods**

- **Diversify Your Intake**: Regularly introduce new fruits, vegetables, whole grains, and protein sources to your diet.
- **Seasonal Adjustments**: Eat seasonally for a natural variety in your diet throughout the year.

2. **Fine-Tuning Macronutrient Ratios**

- **Balance of Proteins, Carbs, and Fats**: Adjust the ratios of macronutrients based on your energy needs, activity levels, and health goals.
- **Consider Food Quality**: Focus on the quality of macronutrients - favoring complex carbs, lean proteins, and healthy fats.

3. **Managing Portion Sizes**

- **Adjust Portions as Needed**: Depending on your activity level and metabolic needs, increase or decrease portion sizes.
- **Use Smaller Plates**: To control portion sizes, use smaller dishes as a simple visual cue.

4. **Listening to Hunger and Fullness Cues**

- **Mindful Eating**: Eat slowly and pay attention to your body's hunger and fullness signals.
- **Avoid Emotional Eating**: Try to eat based on physical need rather than emotional cues.

5. **Hydration**

- **Monitor Water Intake**: Ensure adequate water intake, which can affect digestion and overall body function.
- **Balance with Other Beverages**: Limit high-sugar or caffeinated drinks, opting for herbal teas or infused water.

6. **Experimentation and Flexibility**

- **Try Elimination Diets**: Temporarily eliminate certain foods to identify sensitivities or adverse effects.
- **Be Open to Change**: Stay flexible and open to making changes as your body and lifestyle evolve.

## Conclusion

Adjusting your diet as needed is a crucial aspect of maintaining a pH-balanced diet. It involves being in tune with your body, understanding your health goals, and being willing to make changes for optimal health. Regularly revisiting and revising your diet ensures that it continues to meet your nutritional needs and support your overall well-being. The journey to a balanced diet is ongoing, and embracing flexibility and mindfulness in your dietary choices is key to long-term success.

## Chapter 6: Beyond Diet – Lifestyle and Environmental Factors

### Lifestyle Habits for Optimal pH Balance

### Exercise, sleep, and stress management

A pH-balanced diet is most effective when combined with a holistic lifestyle approach that includes regular exercise, adequate sleep, and effective stress management. These elements work synergistically to enhance overall health and well-being. This chapter delves into the importance of these lifestyle factors and offers practical advice for integrating them into your daily routine.

### Exercise and Physical Activity

Regular physical activity is crucial for maintaining a healthy pH balance in the body, as it helps in the elimination of acids through respiration and perspiration.

1. **Types of Exercise**:
   - **Cardiovascular Activities**: Running, brisk walking, cycling, and swimming help increase lung capacity and efficiency, aiding in acid elimination.
   - **Strength Training**: Builds muscle mass, which can buffer acids in the body.
   - **Flexibility and Balance Exercises**: Yoga and Pilates improve circulation and organ function, contributing to better pH regulation.
2. **Regular Routine**:
   - Aim for at least 150 minutes of moderate aerobic activity or 75 minutes of vigorous activity per week.
   - Include muscle-strengthening activities on two or more days a week.
3. **Exercise and Alkalinity**:
   - Post-exercise, consume alkaline-forming foods like fruits and vegetables to replenish and balance pH levels.

## Sleep and Its Role in pH Balance

Quality sleep is vital for the body's restorative processes, which are crucial for maintaining pH balance.

1. **Adequate Sleep Duration**:
   - Adults should aim for 7-9 hours of sleep per night.
   - Consistent sleep and wake times aid in regulating the body's internal clock.
2. **Sleep Environment**:
   - Create a restful environment, free from electronic devices, and maintain a comfortable temperature.
   - Consider relaxation techniques like reading or meditation before bed.
3. **Impact of Poor Sleep**:
   - Lack of sleep can lead to stress and hormonal imbalances, which may affect the body's ability to maintain pH balance.

## Stress Management and pH Balance

Stress can significantly impact the body's pH levels, as it leads to the production of acid-forming hormones like cortisol.

1. **Identification of Stressors**:
   - Recognize personal stress triggers and understand their effects on your health and dietary choices.
2. **Effective Stress-Relief Techniques**:
   - **Mindfulness and Meditation**: Practices like meditation, deep breathing exercises, and mindfulness can reduce stress levels.
   - **Physical Activity**: Regular exercise is an effective stress reliever.
   - **Hobbies and Leisure Activities**: Engage in activities you enjoy, such as reading, gardening, or painting.
3. **Balanced Lifestyle**:
   - Allocate time for relaxation and self-care.
   - Ensure a balance between work, leisure, and social activities.

**Integrating Exercise, Sleep, and Stress Management**

- Create a daily schedule that includes time for physical activity, relaxation, and sufficient sleep.
- Make gradual changes to incorporate these practices into your lifestyle.
- Be patient and persistent, as developing new habits takes time.

**Conclusion**

Integrating regular exercise, ensuring adequate sleep, and managing stress are essential components of a holistic approach to maintaining a pH-balanced lifestyle.

These practices not only contribute to better physical health but also enhance mental well-being, creating a positive feedback loop that supports your dietary efforts. As you continue to develop and refine your lifestyle choices, remember that balance is key in every aspect of health and wellness. The final chapter will summarize the key principles of maintaining a pH-balanced lifestyle and provide concluding thoughts on embracing this holistic approach.

## Hydration and its role in pH balance

Hydration plays a pivotal role in maintaining pH balance in the body. Water is essential for almost every bodily function, including the regulation of pH levels. This chapter delves into the importance of hydration in maintaining pH balance and offers practical advice for incorporating proper hydration into your daily routine.

### Understanding the Importance of Hydration

Water is crucial for diluting and eliminating waste products from the body. These waste products can be acidic, and their efficient removal is vital for maintaining the body's natural pH balance.

### 1. Water as a Natural pH Regulator

- **Dilution of Acids**: Water helps dilute the concentration of acids in the body, particularly in the bloodstream and kidneys.
- **Elimination of Waste**: Through urination, sweating, and respiration, water aids in the elimination of acidic waste products.
- **Transport of Nutrients**: Adequate hydration ensures efficient transport of nutrients, many of which are essential for maintaining pH balance.

### 2. How Much Water Should You Drink?

- **General Guidelines**: The common recommendation is 8-10 glasses of water per day, but this can vary based on individual factors like weight, climate, and activity level.
- **Listen to Your Body**: Pay attention to thirst signals and urine color (pale yellow is ideal) as indicators of hydration status.

### 3. Impact of Dehydration

- **pH Imbalance**: Dehydration can lead to the accumulation of acids in the body, disrupting pH balance.
- **Health Consequences**: Chronic dehydration can affect kidney function, energy levels, and overall health.

**Incorporating Hydration into Your Daily Routine**

1. **Start the Day with Water**: Begin your day with a glass of water to kickstart hydration and digestion.
2. **Carry a Water Bottle**: Having water on hand at all times encourages regular drinking.
3. **Set Reminders**: Use reminders or apps to prompt regular water intake throughout the day.

**The Role of Beverages in Hydration and pH Balance**

Not all beverages contribute equally to hydration and pH balance. Some can be dehydrating or acidic.

1. **Alkaline Water**: Some people opt for alkaline water, which has a higher pH than regular tap water. While research on its benefits is ongoing, it may contribute to maintaining pH balance.
2. **Limit Caffeinated and Alcoholic Beverages**: These can be dehydrating and may contribute to acidity in the body. Moderation is key.
3. **Herbal Teas**: A good alternative to plain water, many herbal teas are hydrating and have a neutral or alkaline effect on the body's pH.

**Hydration in Different Conditions**

1. **Exercise**: Increase water intake during and after exercise to compensate for fluid loss through sweating.
2. **Hot Weather**: In warm climates or during summer, the body loses more water through sweat, necessitating increased fluid intake.
3. **Illness**: During illness, especially with fever, diarrhea, or vomiting, hydration becomes even more critical.

**Conclusion**

Hydration is a cornerstone of maintaining a balanced pH in the body. Adequate water intake ensures the efficient dilution and elimination of acidic waste, aiding in overall health and well-being.

By incorporating hydration strategies into your daily life, you can support your body's natural pH regulation processes. As you continue to explore the principles of a pH-balanced lifestyle, remember that consistent hydration is a simple yet powerful tool for maintaining optimal health.

## Environmental Influences

### External factors affecting body pH

While diet plays a crucial role in maintaining the body's pH balance, several external factors can also significantly impact it. Understanding and managing these factors are essential for maintaining optimal health. This chapter explores various external influences on body pH and offers strategies to mitigate their effects.

### Environmental Toxins

Pollutants and chemicals in the environment can affect the body's acid-alkaline balance.

1. **Air Pollution**:
    - Inhaling polluted air can introduce acidic compounds into the body, affecting lung and overall health.
    - **Mitigation**: Use air purifiers indoors and wear masks in highly polluted areas.
2. **Chemical Exposure**:
    - Exposure to chemicals in cleaning products, pesticides, and plastics can contribute to acidity.
    - **Mitigation**: Use natural cleaning products and minimize the use of plastic.

### Stress and Emotional Well-being

Stress can lead to the production of acid-forming hormones like cortisol and adrenaline.

1. **Chronic Stress**:
    - Long-term stress can disrupt hormonal balance, leading to increased acidity.
    - **Mitigation**: Engage in stress-reduction activities like meditation, yoga, or deep breathing exercises.
2. **Emotional Health**:
    - Negative emotions such as anger and fear can create a biochemical response, increasing acidity.
    - **Mitigation**: Seek counseling or therapy to manage emotional challenges effectively.

## Physical Activity Levels

Exercise impacts acid-base balance in both short-term and long-term ways.

1. **Intense Exercise**:
   - High-intensity workouts can produce lactic acid, temporarily increasing body acidity.
   - **Mitigation**: Balance high-intensity workouts with moderate activities and ensure proper hydration.
2. **Sedentary Lifestyle**:
   - Lack of physical activity can impair metabolic processes, influencing pH balance.
   - **Mitigation**: Incorporate regular physical activity into your routine, aiming for a mix of cardiovascular, strength, and flexibility exercises.

## Medications and Supplements

Certain medications and supplements can affect the body's pH levels.

1. **Prescription Drugs**:
   - Some medications, like diuretics or corticosteroids, can impact kidney function and pH balance.
   - **Mitigation**: Consult with healthcare providers about the pH effects of prescribed medications and explore alternatives if necessary.
2. **Supplements**:
   - Overuse of supplements, particularly acid-forming ones like high doses of vitamin C or certain protein powders, can alter pH levels.
   - **Mitigation**: Take supplements as recommended and choose those that support pH balance.

## Hydration and Fluid Intake

The type and amount of fluids consumed can influence acid-alkaline balance.

1. **Inadequate Water Intake**:
   - Not drinking enough water can concentrate body fluids, increasing acidity.
   - **Mitigation**: Ensure adequate hydration by drinking water throughout the day.
2. **Acidic Beverages**:
   - Consumption of high volumes of acidic drinks like coffee, alcohol, or sugary sodas can impact pH.
   - **Mitigation**: Limit intake of these beverages and opt for more alkaline or neutral options like herbal teas or water.

## Sleep Patterns

Sleep quality and quantity can indirectly affect body pH.

1. **Poor Sleep Quality**:
   - Lack of restorative sleep can lead to stress and hormonal imbalances, affecting pH balance.
   - **Mitigation**: Establish a regular sleep routine and create a conducive sleep environment.

## Conclusion

External factors play a significant role in influencing the body's pH balance. By being aware of these influences and adopting strategies to mitigate their impact, individuals can better maintain their overall health and pH balance. A holistic approach that considers both dietary and lifestyle factors is key to managing body pH effectively.

**How to mitigate negative influences**

Maintaining a pH-balanced lifestyle involves not only focusing on diet and exercise but also addressing and mitigating various external factors that can negatively influence your body's pH. This chapter explores practical strategies to counteract these negative influences, ensuring a holistic approach to maintaining optimal health.

## 1. Reducing Exposure to Environmental Toxins

Environmental toxins can significantly disrupt the body's acid-alkaline balance. Minimizing exposure is crucial:

- **Air Quality**: Utilize air purifiers in your home and office to reduce the inhalation of pollutants.
- **Water Filtration**: Use water filters to remove potential contaminants from your drinking water.
- **Natural Products**: Opt for natural, eco-friendly cleaning and personal care products to reduce chemical exposure.
- **Organic Foods**: Whenever possible, choose organic produce to avoid pesticide residues.

## 2. Managing Stress Effectively

Chronic stress leads to an increase in acid-forming hormones like cortisol. Effective stress management is key:

- **Regular Relaxation Practices**: Incorporate relaxation techniques such as yoga, meditation, or deep breathing exercises into your daily routine.
- **Time Management**: Organize your schedule to reduce overwhelm and allow time for rest and relaxation.
- **Seek Support**: Don't hesitate to seek professional help if stress becomes unmanageable.

## 3. Ensuring Adequate Physical Activity

Both excessive and insufficient physical activity can affect pH balance:

- **Balanced Exercise Regimen**: Combine cardio, strength training, and flexibility exercises for a balanced workout routine.
- **Post-Workout Recovery**: Include alkaline-forming foods in your post-workout meal to neutralize any excess acid produced during exercise.
- **Regular Movement**: Incorporate movement into your day, especially if you have a sedentary job, to stimulate circulation and metabolism.

## 4. Mindful Medication and Supplement Use

Certain medications and supplements can disrupt pH balance:

- **Consult Healthcare Professionals**: Regularly review your medications and supplements with your healthcare provider, focusing on their impact on pH balance.
- **Natural Alternatives**: Where possible, explore natural alternatives to conventional medications.
- **Responsible Supplement Use**: Only use supplements that are necessary and beneficial for your health, avoiding excessive or unnecessary consumption.

## 5. Prioritizing Hydration

Proper hydration is essential for maintaining pH balance:

- **Adequate Water Intake**: Aim to drink at least 8-10 glasses of water daily.
- **Limit Acidic Beverages**: Reduce consumption of caffeinated, sugary, and alcoholic beverages.
- **Herbal Teas**: Incorporate herbal teas, which can be beneficial for pH balance and hydration.

## 6. Healthy Sleep Habits

Quality sleep is crucial for overall health and pH balance:

- **Consistent Sleep Schedule**: Maintain a regular sleep routine to enhance sleep quality.
- **Sleep-Inducing Environment**: Create a restful sleeping environment, free from electronic devices and distractions.
- **Sleep Hygiene Practices**: Engage in calming activities before bed, such as reading or taking a warm bath.

## 7. Nutritional Balance

Balanced nutrition is the cornerstone of maintaining a healthy pH level:

- **Diverse Diet**: Ensure your diet includes a wide range of nutrients from various food groups, focusing on a balance of acidic and alkaline foods.
- **Portion Control**: Be mindful of portion sizes, especially for acid-forming foods.
- **Mindful Eating**: Pay attention to how different foods affect your body and adjust your diet accordingly.

## 8. Community and Social Support

Having a supportive community can positively impact your ability to maintain a pH-balanced lifestyle:

- **Share Your Goals**: Communicate your health goals with friends and family to gain their support.
- **Join Supportive Groups**: Consider joining groups or forums that focus on pH-balanced living for motivation and advice.

## Conclusion

Mitigating the negative influences on pH balance requires a multifaceted approach that includes environmental considerations, stress management, physical activity, careful use of medications and supplements, proper hydration, good sleep hygiene, and nutritional balance. By addressing these areas, you can create a conducive environment for maintaining optimal pH levels, leading to improved health and well-being.

# Conclusion

## The Journey to pH Balance

### Recap of key points

As we conclude our exploration of maintaining a pH-balanced diet, it's beneficial to recapitulate the key points that have been discussed throughout this guide. This chapter provides a summary of the essential principles and practices for achieving and sustaining a pH-balanced lifestyle.

### Understanding pH Balance

- **pH Basics**: pH is a measure of how acidic or alkaline a substance is, on a scale from 0 (highly acidic) to 14 (highly alkaline), with 7 being neutral.
- **Body pH**: The human body strives to maintain a slightly alkaline pH level, especially in the blood, for optimal functioning.

### Dietary Focus

- **Acidic and Alkaline Foods**: A balance of acidic (meat, grains, dairy) and alkaline foods (fruits, vegetables, nuts) is crucial.
- **Importance of Variety**: A diverse diet ensures a broad spectrum of nutrients, supporting overall health and pH balance.

### Role of Lifestyle Factors

- **Hydration**: Adequate water intake is essential for diluting and eliminating acidic waste from the body.
- **Exercise**: Regular physical activity helps in maintaining a balanced metabolism and aids in detoxification.
- **Stress Management**: Managing stress is vital as it can affect hormonal balance and, consequently, body pH.
- **Sleep**: Quality sleep supports the body's regulatory processes, including pH balance.

### Overcoming Challenges

- **Identifying Triggers**: Recognize and manage personal triggers like emotional eating, stress, or certain food cravings.
- **Adapting to Changes**: Be flexible and willing to adjust your diet and lifestyle as your body, environment, and circumstances change.

## Health Benefits

- **Preventive Health**: A pH-balanced diet can contribute to bone health, muscle preservation, improved digestion, and reduced risk of chronic diseases.
- **Overall Wellness**: Beyond physical health, balancing dietary pH can enhance mental and emotional well-being.

## Practical Strategies

- **Meal Planning**: Plan meals to include a balance of acidic and alkaline foods, and prepare in advance to ease dietary adherence.
- **Mindful Eating**: Pay attention to how foods affect your body and adjust your eating habits accordingly.
- **Supportive Environment**: Create a supportive environment for a pH-balanced lifestyle, including kitchen setup, social interactions, and stress-free spaces.

## Common Misconceptions

- **Food pH vs. Effect on Body**: The pH value of food in its natural state can be different from its effect on the body's pH after metabolism.
- **Absolute Avoidance**: It is not about completely avoiding acidic foods, but about finding a harmonious balance in your diet.

## Final Thoughts

Achieving a pH-balanced diet is a dynamic process that involves mindful eating, understanding of nutritional science, and a holistic approach to lifestyle changes. It requires patience, persistence, and a willingness to learn and adapt.

Remember, the goal is not perfection but progress towards a healthier, more balanced way of living. By embracing the principles outlined in this guide, you can embark on a journey towards enhanced health and well-being, supported by a diet and lifestyle that promote optimal pH balance.

## Encouragement for ongoing wellness

Embarking on a journey to maintain a pH-balanced diet and a healthy lifestyle is commendable. It's a path that leads to enhanced well-being, vitality, and longevity. However, like any journey, it can have its challenges and moments of doubt. This chapter is dedicated to providing encouragement for ongoing wellness, underscoring the importance of perseverance, self-compassion, and continuous learning in this lifelong journey.

### Celebrating Small Victories

1. **Acknowledge Progress**: No matter how small, every step towards a healthier lifestyle is a victory. Celebrate these moments.
2. **Reflect on Improvements**: Regularly reflect on how changes in diet and lifestyle have positively impacted your health and well-being.

### Cultivating a Positive Mindset

1. **Stay Optimistic**: Maintain a positive outlook on your health journey. Optimism can be a powerful tool in overcoming challenges.
2. **Embrace Setbacks as Learning Opportunities**: Understand that setbacks are part of the journey. Use them to learn and grow.

### Building a Supportive Community

1. **Seek Support**: Surround yourself with people who support and encourage your wellness goals. This could be friends, family, or online communities.
2. **Share Your Journey**: Sharing your experiences can not only help others but also reinforce your commitment to wellness.

### Continual Learning and Adaptation

1. **Stay Informed**: Keep up-to-date with the latest research and information on nutrition and wellness.
2. **Be Open to Change**: As new information emerges, be willing to adapt your approach to wellness.

### Balancing Wellness with Everyday Life

1. **Integrate, Don't Isolate**: Incorporate wellness into your daily life instead of viewing it as separate. Find ways to blend healthy habits with your routine.
2. **Flexible Approach**: Be flexible in your approach to diet and exercise. Rigidity can lead to frustration and burnout.

## Mindful and Intuitive Eating

1. **Listen to Your Body**: Tune into your body's cues. Eat when you're hungry, stop when you're full, and be mindful of what your body needs.
2. **Enjoy Your Food**: Take pleasure in eating. Savor flavors, textures, and the experience of nourishing your body.

## Regular Self-Care and Relaxation

1. **Prioritize Self-Care**: Regularly engage in activities that relax and rejuvenate you, whether it's a hobby, meditation, or a walk in nature.
2. **Balance Activity with Rest**: Alongside physical activity, ensure you get enough rest. Rest is a crucial component of a holistic wellness approach.

## Setting Realistic Goals and Expectations

1. **Realistic Goals**: Set achievable goals that motivate you without causing undue stress.
2. **Patience with the Process**: Understand that progress can be slow and that's perfectly okay.

## Conclusion

Maintaining ongoing wellness is a dynamic and continuous process. It requires commitment, but it should also be a journey of joy and discovery. Celebrate your successes, learn from the challenges, and embrace the journey with a positive and open mindset.

Remember, the ultimate goal is not just to achieve a certain state of health but to enjoy a richer, fuller life. Your journey to wellness is unique and deeply personal, and every step you take towards this goal is a testament to your commitment to living your best life.

**Appendices**

**Food pH Charts and References**

This section provides comprehensive charts categorizing common foods based on their pH levels and potential impact on the body's pH balance. These references can be a helpful guide in making informed dietary choices for maintaining a pH-balanced diet.

**Highly Acidic Foods (pH 0-4.5)**

- **Fruits**: Lemons (pH 2-3), Limes (pH 2-2.8), Oranges (pH 3-4)
- **Berries**: Strawberries (pH 3-3.5), Blueberries (pH 3-3.2)
- **Vinegars**: Apple Cider Vinegar (pH 2.5-3), White Vinegar (pH 2.4)
- **Fermented Foods**: Sauerkraut (pH 3.1-3.6), Yogurt (pH 3.5-4.5)

**Moderately Acidic Foods (pH 4.6-5.5)**

- **Dairy Products**: Cow's Milk (pH 4.6-4.8), Cheese (pH around 5)
- **Grains**: White Bread (pH 5-5.5), Whole Wheat Bread (pH 5.5)

**Neutral Foods (pH 6-7)**

- **Fats and Oils**: Olive Oil (pH 7), Butter (pH 6.1-6.4)

**Mildly Alkaline Foods (pH 7.1-8)**

- **Vegetables**: Spinach (pH 7.2-7.5), Cucumbers (pH 7.1-7.6)
- **Fruits**: Bananas (pH 7.1-7.5), Avocados (pH 7.5-7.8)

**Highly Alkaline Foods (pH 8.1-9)**

- **Leafy Greens**: Kale (pH 8.5), Swiss Chard (pH 8.3)
- **Root Vegetables**: Carrots (pH 8.1-8.3), Beets (pH 8.2-8.5)

**Special Considerations**

- Citrus fruits like lemons and limes, though acidic in nature, have an alkalizing effect after digestion due to their mineral content.
- Dairy products, generally considered acid-forming, are high in protein and phosphorus, contributing to their acidifying effect in the body.

**Food pH Chart: Highly Acidic Foods (pH 0-4.5)**

This chart lists 30 foods that fall into the highly acidic category, along with their approximate pH values. These foods, while diverse in nature, share the common characteristic of being highly acidic.

1. **Lemons**: pH 2-3
2. **Limes**: pH 2-2.8
3. **Grapefruits**: pH 3-3.5
4. **Cranberries**: pH 2.3-2.5
5. **Pickles**: pH 3.2-3.5
6. **Sauerkraut**: pH 3.1-3.6
7. **Apple Cider Vinegar**: pH 2.5-3
8. **White Vinegar**: pH 2.4
9. **Yogurt**: pH 3.5-4.5
10. **Sour Cream**: pH 4.0-4.5
11. **Buttermilk**: pH 4.4-4.8
12. **Black Coffee**: pH 4.0-5.0
13. **Wine**: pH 3.0-3.5
14. **Beer**: pH 3.0-4.0
15. **Soft Drinks**: pH 2.5-4.0
16. **Plums**: pH 2.8-3.0
17. **Pomegranates**: pH 2.9-3.2
18. **Raspberries**: pH 3.2-3.5
19. **Blackberries**: pH 3.5-4.0
20. **Cherries**: pH 3.2-4.0
21. **Pineapples**: pH 3.2-4.0
22. **Green Apples**: pH 3.0-4.0
23. **Blueberries**: pH 3.1-3.4
24. **Oranges**: pH 3.0-4.0
25. **Peaches**: pH 3.4-4.5
26. **Kiwi Fruit**: pH 3.1-4.1
27. **Strawberries**: pH 3-3.5
28. **Ketchup**: pH 3.9-4.0
29. **Mustard**: pH 3.5-4.0
30. **Tomatoes**: pH 4.3-4.9

## Food pH Chart: Moderately Acidic Foods (pH 4.6-5.5)

This chart provides a list of 30 foods that are categorized as moderately acidic, featuring their approximate pH values. These foods have a mild to moderate acidic nature.

1. **Cow's Milk**: pH 4.6-4.8
2. **Cheddar Cheese**: pH 5.1-5.5
3. **Cottage Cheese**: pH 4.5-5.0
4. **Sour Dough Bread**: pH 4.4-5.0
5. **White Bread**: pH 5.0-5.5
6. **Whole Wheat Bread**: pH 4.9-5.5
7. **Brown Rice**: pH 5.0-5.5
8. **Wild Rice**: pH 5.0-5.5
9. **Oats**: pH 4.9-5.5
10. **Lentils**: pH 5.0-5.5
11. **Chickpeas**: pH 4.6-5.0
12. **Corn**: pH 4.5-5.0
13. **Green Peas**: pH 4.8-5.5
14. **Honey**: pH 4.5-5.0
15. **Maple Syrup**: pH 5.0-5.5
16. **Balsamic Vinegar**: pH 4.5-5.0
17. **Soy Sauce**: pH 4.9-5.5
18. **Black Tea (Brewed)**: pH 4.9-5.5
19. **Peanuts**: pH 4.8-5.0
20. **Cashews**: pH 4.9-5.5
21. **Pistachios**: pH 4.9-5.5
22. **Sunflower Seeds**: pH 5.0-5.5
23. **Walnuts**: pH 4.6-5.0
24. **Almonds**: pH 4.6-5.0
25. **Pumpkin Seeds**: pH 5.0-5.5
26. **Olives**: pH 4.6-5.0
27. **Cranberry Juice**: pH 4.5-5.0
28. **Apple Juice**: pH 4.0-4.5
29. **Grape Juice**: pH 4.5-5.0
30. **Mango**: pH 4.6-5.0

**Note**:

- The pH values listed are approximate and can vary based on factors such as preparation, processing, and ripeness.
- Moderately acidic foods can be part of a balanced diet, but it's important to consume them in moderation, especially for individuals who are managing acid reflux or aiming for a more alkaline diet.
- Combining these foods with alkaline-forming foods can help balance their acidic nature.

## Food pH Chart: Neutral Foods (pH 6-7)

This chart lists 30 foods that are considered to have a neutral pH, falling in the range of 6 to 7. These foods are neither significantly acidic nor alkaline and can be important components of a balanced diet.

1. **Butter**: pH 6.1-6.4
2. **Margarine**: pH 6.5
3. **Whole Cow's Milk**: pH 6.5-6.7
4. **Skim Milk**: pH 6.7
5. **Heavy Cream**: pH 6.5
6. **Eggs (Whole)**: pH 6.0-6.5
7. **Yogurt (Plain)**: pH 6.5
8. **Natural Cheese (Most varieties)**: pH 6.0-7.0
9. **Whey (Fresh)**: pH 6.4-6.6
10. **White Rice**: pH 6.0-6.7
11. **Brown Rice**: pH 6.2-6.7
12. **Quinoa**: pH 6.0-6.5
13. **Basmati Rice**: pH 6.0-6.5
14. **Barley**: pH 6.0-6.5
15. **Oatmeal**: pH 6.0-7.0
16. **Almond Milk**: pH 6.0-7.0
17. **Soy Milk**: pH 6.0-7.0
18. **Rice Milk**: pH 6.5-7.0
19. **Chicken Breast (Cooked)**: pH 6.0-6.5
20. **Turkey (Cooked)**: pH 6.0-6.5
21. **Pasta (Cooked)**: pH 6.0-6.5
22. **White Bread (Fresh)**: pH 6.0-6.5
23. **Whole Wheat Bread (Fresh)**: pH 6.0-6.5
24. **Beef (Cooked)**: pH 6.0-6.5
25. **Pork (Cooked)**: pH 6.0-6.5
26. **Veal (Cooked)**: pH 6.0-6.5
27. **Fish (Fresh, Cooked)**: pH 6.0-6.5
28. **Honey**: pH 6.0-6.5
29. **Maple Syrup**: pH 6.0-7.0
30. **Canola Oil**: pH 6.0-7.0

**Note**:

- The pH values listed are approximate and can vary depending on factors such as processing, preparation, and storage conditions.
- Neutral foods are typically well-tolerated and can be a safe choice for people with sensitivities to highly acidic or alkaline foods.
- Including a variety of neutral foods in your diet can contribute to a well-rounded and nutritionally balanced eating plan.

**Food pH Chart: Mildly Alkaline Foods (pH 7.1-8)**

This chart features 30 foods that fall within the mildly alkaline range, with their approximate pH values. Incorporating these foods can help balance the overall pH levels in your diet.

1. **Spinach**: pH 7.2-7.5
2. **Kale**: pH 7.3-7.5
3. **Broccoli**: pH 7.1-7.3
4. **Cauliflower**: pH 7.2-7.4
5. **Cucumbers**: pH 7.1-7.6
6. **Celery**: pH 7.2-7.4
7. **Carrots**: pH 7.1-7.3
8. **Sweet Potatoes**: pH 7.2-7.5
9. **Red Bell Peppers**: pH 7.1-7.3
10. **Zucchini**: pH 7.2-7.5
11. **Green Beans**: pH 7.1-7.5
12. **Lettuce**: pH 7.1-7.2
13. **Bananas**: pH 7.1-7.5
14. **Avocados**: pH 7.5-7.8
15. **Cantaloupe**: pH 7.1-7.5
16. **Mangoes**: pH 7.1-7.5
17. **Papayas**: pH 7.2-7.5
18. **Kiwifruit**: pH 7.1-7.5
19. **Apples**: pH 7.1-7.4
20. **Pears**: pH 7.1-7.5
21. **Apricots**: pH 7.1-7.4
22. **Peaches**: pH 7.1-7.4
23. **Nectarines**: pH 7.1-7.5
24. **Almonds**: pH 7.1-8.0
25. **Chestnuts**: pH 7.5-8.0
26. **Tofu**: pH 7.1-7.5
27. **Soybeans**: pH 7.1-7.5
28. **Quinoa**: pH 7.1-7.4
29. **Millet**: pH 7.1-7.5
30. **Herbal Teas**: pH 7.1-7.5

**Note:**

- The pH values of these foods are approximate and can vary based on factors like ripeness, preparation, and brand.
- While mildly alkaline, these foods can contribute significantly to balancing the body's overall pH when included as part of a varied diet.
- Consuming a mix of mildly alkaline foods alongside slightly acidic and neutral foods can help achieve a well-rounded and nutritionally diverse diet.

**Food pH Chart: Highly Alkaline Foods (pH 8.1-9)**

This chart enumerates 30 foods that are categorized as highly alkaline, with their approximate pH values. These foods can significantly contribute to increasing the body's alkalinity.

1. **Baking Soda**: pH 9.0
2. **Lemon Water**: pH 8.5 (once metabolized)
3. **Seaweed**: pH 8.0-9.0
4. **Kale**: pH 8.5
5. **Spinach**: pH 8.5
6. **Swiss Chard**: pH 8.3
7. **Watercress**: pH 8.5
8. **Beet Greens**: pH 8.5
9. **Dandelion Greens**: pH 8.5
10. **Mustard Greens**: pH 8.5
11. **Cabbage**: pH 8.2-8.5
12. **Wheatgrass**: pH 8.5
13. **Barley Grass**: pH 8.5
14. **Spirulina**: pH 8.5
15. **Chlorella**: pH 8.5
16. **Parsley**: pH 8.5
17. **Cucumber**: pH 8.5
18. **Broccoli**: pH 8.5
19. **Celery**: pH 8.5
20. **Carrots**: pH 8.5
21. **Green Beans**: pH 8.5
22. **Lettuce**: pH 8.5
23. **Zucchini**: pH 8.5
24. **Asparagus**: pH 8.5
25. **Radicchio**: pH 8.5
26. **Basil**: pH 8.5
27. **Coriander**: pH 8.5
28. **Herbal Teas (e.g., Chamomile, Mint)**: pH 8.5
29. **Artichokes**: pH 8.5
30. **Lemon Juice**: pH 8.5 (once metabolized)

**Note**:

- The pH values listed for these foods are approximate and can vary based on factors like ripeness, preparation, and cultivation.
- Despite their initial acidic nature, some foods like lemon water and lemon juice become highly alkaline once metabolized in the body.
- Consuming a variety of highly alkaline foods can help neutralize excess acids in the diet, promoting a balanced pH level within the body. However, it's important to maintain a balanced and varied diet for overall nutritional health.

## Glossary

This glossary provides definitions for key terms used throughout the book, offering readers a deeper understanding of concepts related to pH balance and nutrition.

1. **Acidosis**: A condition characterized by an excess of acid in the body fluids, typically marked by a lower-than-normal blood pH.
2. **Alkaline Diet**: A diet that focuses on foods believed to produce less acid within the body, typically emphasizing fruits, vegetables, nuts, and legumes.
3. **Alkalosis**: A condition resulting from a decrease in the hydrogen ion concentration of the blood, leading to an increase in pH above the normal range.
4. **Antioxidants**: Compounds found in food that can prevent or slow damage to cells caused by free radicals. Common in fruits and vegetables.
5. **Bicarbonate**: A primary component of the alkaline buffer system in the blood, helping to maintain pH balance by neutralizing acids.
6. **Buffer Systems**: Mechanisms in the blood and cells that maintain pH balance by neutralizing excess acids or bases.
7. **Electrolytes**: Minerals in the body (like sodium, potassium, and calcium) that maintain the balance of fluids and pH.
8. **Fermentation**: A metabolic process that produces chemical changes in organic substrates through the action of enzymes, often resulting in acidic by-products.
9. **Hydration**: The process of providing an adequate amount of liquid to bodily tissues.
10. **Macro-nutrients**: Nutrients required in large amounts for normal growth and development, including carbohydrates, proteins, and fats.
11. **Metabolism**: The set of life-sustaining chemical reactions in organisms, including converting food to energy, constructing cellular components, and eliminating waste products.
12. **Micro-nutrients**: Essential nutrients, such as vitamins and minerals, required in smaller amounts for proper body functioning.
13. **pH**: A scale used to specify the acidity or alkalinity of an aqueous solution. Ranges from 0 (highly acidic) to 14 (highly alkaline), with 7 being neutral.
14. **Potential Renal Acid Load (PRAL)**: A measure used to estimate the production of acid in the kidneys after the body metabolizes food.
15. **Probiotics**: Live microorganisms, typically bacteria, that provide health benefits when consumed by improving or restoring gut flora.
16. **Processed Foods**: Foods that have been altered from their original state, often through the addition of ingredients, for convenience, shelf stability, or flavor enhancement.
17. **Whole Foods**: Foods that are minimally processed, refined, or handled, making them as close to their natural form as possible.